Cocaine-Exposed
Infants

Drugs, Health, and Social Policy Series

Edited by James A. Inciardi
University of Delaware

About This Series . . .

The Sage **Drugs, Health, and Social Policy Series** provides students and professionals in the fields of substance abuse, AIDS, public health, and criminal justice access to current research, programs, and policy issues particular to their specialties. Each year, four new volumes will focus on a topic of national significance.

Cocaine-Exposed Infants

Social, Legal, and Public Health Issues

James A. Inciardi
Hilary L. Surratt
Christine A. Saum

Drugs, Health, and Social Policy Series
Volume 5

SAGE Publications
International Educational and Professional Publisher
Thousand Oaks   London   New Delhi

For information address:

SAGE Publications, Inc.
2455 Teller Road
Thousand Oaks, California 91320
E-mail: order@sagepub.com

SAGE Publications Ltd.
6 Bonhill Street
London EC2A 4PU
United Kingdom

SAGE Publications India Pvt. Ltd.
M-32 Market
Greater Kailash I
New Delhi 110 048 India

Printed in the United States of America

Library of Congress Cataloging-in-Publication Data

Inciardi, James A.
    Cocaine-exposed infants: social, legal, and public health issues
/ James A. Inciardi, Hilary L. Surratt, Christine A. Saum.
      p. cm. -- (Drugs, health, and social policy series; 5)
    Includes bibliographical references and indexes.
    ISBN 0-8039-7086-2 (cloth). — ISBN 0-8039-7087-0 (pbk.)
    1. Drug abuse in pregnancy. 2. Cocaine—Toxicology. 3. Fetus-
-Effect of drugs on. 4. Children of prenatal substance abuse.
5. Drug abuse in pregnancy—Government policy—United States.
I. Surratt, Hilary L. II. Saum, Christine A. III. Title.
RG580.D76I53 1997
618.3'268—dc21   97-4589

This book is printed on acid-free paper.

97 98 99 00 01 02 10 9 8 7 6 5 4 3 2 1

Acquiring Editor:	C. Terry Hendrix
Editorial Assistant:	Dale Grenfell
Production Editor:	Sherrise M. Purdum
Production Assistant:	Karen Wiley
Typesetter & Designer:	Yang-hee Syn Maresca
Indexer:	Juniee Oneida

Contents

Preface

Only three decades ago, the prevailing image of the womb was that of a time capsule with a short lease, relatively impermeable to circulating drugs or toxicants. The mother's body was considered an altruistic reservoir, prepared to sacrifice itself to the fetus's sustenance.

—Needleman and Bellinger (1994, p. ix)

Although it is now known that the placenta does not always act as a protective barrier between mother and child, many women remain unaware that drugs can indeed cross the placental wall, and that cocaine in particular readily passes from maternal to fetal circulation (Dixon, 1994; Schneider, Griffith, & Chasnoff, 1989). Moreover, it has only been since the tragedy of thalidomide-poisoned fetuses in the early 1960s that the use of drugs during pregnancy began to receive close attention.[1] In subsequent years, alcohol use during pregnancy garnered considerable recognition as researchers verified the long-suspected connections between the drinking patterns of alcoholic women and the incidence of retardation and birth defects among their offspring (see Jones, Smith, Ulleland, & Streissguth, 1973).

By the late 1970s, the use of cocaine became relatively visible in both rural and urban America. Moreover, with the appearance of crack in the 1980s and its apparent epidemic use in numerous inner-city communities, reports of child abuse and neglect by crack-addicted parents were publicized in the national media, as were graphic descriptions of an allegedly growing population of impaired, so-called crack-addicted infants born (and sometimes abandoned) in the nation's hospitals. And as research programs and studies on the effects of fetal exposure to cocaine increased, legislation was passed in a variety of jurisdictions that served to criminalize cocaine and other drug use during pregnancy.

Without question, cocaine is a seductive and dangerous drug, and any form of cocaine use can have a negative impact on the developing fetus. Indeed, there are many associations between cocaine use and negative fetal outcome. Yet, scientific proof of a cause and effect relationship between cocaine use and adverse prenatal and postnatal consequences has been difficult to establish. Part of the problem is that many cocaine-using mothers abuse other illegal drugs, and many consume alcohol and tobacco as well. Another difficulty lies with much of the early research on prenatal cocaine exposure. Many studies had numerous methodological problems, resulting in either tentative or problematic conclusions.

Within this context, it is the intention of this book to present what is currently known about cocaine-exposed infants and to unravel some of the contradictions in the literature. By way of introduction, Chapter 1 provides background information on cocaine and crack and offers some general insights and research findings on drug abuse among women. Chapter 2 addresses the myths and misconceptions about so-called crack babies, as well as the ways that some of the early research on prenatal cocaine abuse served to generalize and mislabel the effects of cocaine exposure. Chapter 3 discusses the effects of prenatal exposure to cocaine on a woman's pregnancy, her developing fetus, infant, and child. Chapter 4 examines the many criminal and civil actions that have been filed against pregnant drug abusers, the constitutionality of punitive state intervention, and the consequences of these actions on public policy and maternal drug use.

No book is written without the assistance of many people. In this regard, there are several of our colleagues who contributed to our preparation of this manuscript: Janice Atchley, Paige Magner, Jill McCorkle, Jane Reynolds, and Sidney Schnoll. For all of their help, we are very thankful.

Note

1. Thalidomide was used extensively as a sleeping medication in the early 1960s. Its use was discontinued when it was discovered to cause severe malformations in the limbs of developing fetuses exposed to the drug during the early stages of pregnancy.

1. Cocaine, Crack, and Women

The cocaine problem in the United States has a relatively short history. Although the chewing of coca had already been in Inca mythology for centuries when the Spanish conquistadors stumbled on the Inca empire in 1531, the abuse of cocaine did not emerge until many hundreds of years later. The discovery of crack cocaine and the initial concerns over cocaine-exposed infants, moreover, date back to little more than a decade ago. Both of these latter phenomena have attracted the focused attention of public health organizations, the media, state and federal legislatures, criminal justice systems, and the general public. Given this, it is the intent of this opening chapter to provide brief overviews of the history of cocaine, patterns of cocaine use, the emergence of crack cocaine, the general health consequences of cocaine (including crack) use, and issues associated with drug use among women in general and cocaine use among women in particular.

Coca and Cocaine

The beginnings of cocaine use and abuse in the United States were intimately tied to both the patent medicine industry and the work of Sigmund Freud during the latter years of the 19th century. As early as the 18th century, patent medicines containing opium were readily available throughout urban and rural America. They were sold in pharmacies, grocery and general stores, at traveling medicine shows, and through the mail. Moreover, they were marketed under such alluring labels as Ayer's Cherry Pectoral, Mrs. Winslow's Soothing Syrup, and Godfrey's Cordial, to name but a few. Many of these remedies were seductively advertised as "painkillers," "cough mixtures," "soothing syrups," "consumption cures," and "women's friends." Others were promoted for the treatment of such varied ailments as diarrhea, dysentery, colds, fever, teething, cholera, rheumatism, pelvic disorders, athlete's foot, and even baldness and cancer (Inciardi, 1992). And with the isolation of morphine as the chief alkaloid of opium in 1803, morphine was soon added to the pharmacopeia of over-the-counter patent medicines and home remedies.

Beyond opium and morphine, the patent-medicine industry branched farther. Although chewing coca leaves for their mild stimulant effects had been a part of Andean culture for perhaps 1,000 years, the practice had never been popular in either Europe or the United States. During the latter part of the 19th century, however, Angelo Mariani of Corsica imported many tons of coca leaves to his native land for the production of what he called *Vin Coca Mariani* (Blejer, 1965, p. 702). It was a mixture of extracts from the coca leaf and wine, and it was an immediate success—having been publicized as a magical beverage that would free the body from fatigue, lift the spirits, and create a lasting sense of well-being.

Vin Coca brought Mr. Mariani immediate wealth and fame, and his success did not go unnoticed by several observers in the United States, including John Styth Pemberton of Atlanta, Georgia. Pemberton had been marketing a number of patent medicines, but noting Mariani's great success, in 1885, he developed a product that he registered as French Wine Coca—Ideal Nerve and Tonic Stimulant. It was originally a medicinal preparation, but the following year, he added an additional ingredient, changed it into a soft drink, and renamed it Coca-Cola (Kahn, 1960).

Although extracts of coca were indeed present in Pemberton's Coca-Cola, the stimulant effects of the drink were at best mild, for after all, the actual amount of cocaine in the leaves was (and remains) quite small—perhaps 1% by weight. Although cocaine in its purest form was first isolated from the coca leaf in 1860, little use was made of the new alkaloid until 1883 when Dr. Theodor Aschenbrandt secured a supply of the drug and issued it to Bavarian soldiers during maneuvers. Aschenbrandt, a German military physician, noted the beneficial effects of cocaine, particularly its ability to suppress fatigue.

Among those who read Aschenbrandt's account with fascination was a struggling young Viennese neurologist, Sigmund Freud. Suffering from chronic fatigue, depression, and various neurotic symptoms, Freud obtained a measure of cocaine and tried it himself. He also offered it to a colleague who was suffering from both a disease of the nervous system and morphine addiction and to a patient with a chronic and painful gastric disorder. Finding the initial results to be quite favorable in all three cases, Freud decided that cocaine was a magical drug. In a letter to his fiancee, Martha Bernays, in 1884, Freud commented on his experiences with cocaine:

> If all goes well I will write an essay on it and I expect it will win its place in therapeutics by the side of morphium and superior to it. I have other hopes and intentions about it. I take very small doses of it regularly against depression and against indigestion, and with the most brilliant success. . . . In short it is only now that I feel that I am a doctor, since I have helped one patient and hope to help more. (Jones, 1953, p. 81)

Freud then pressed the drug onto his friends and colleagues, urging that they use it both for themselves and their patients; he gave it to his sisters and his fiancée and continued to use it himself. By the close of the 1880s, however, Freud and the others who had praised cocaine as an all-purpose wonder drug began to withdraw their support for it in light of an increasing number of reports of compulsive use and undesirable side effects. Yet by 1890, the patent-medicine industry in the United States had also discovered the benefits of the unregulated use of cocaine. The industry quickly added the drug to its reservoir of home remedies, touting it as helpful not only for everything from alcoholism to venereal disease but also as a cure for addiction to other patent medicines. Because the new tonics contained substantial amounts of cocaine, they did indeed make users feel better, at least initially, thus spiriting the patent-medicine industry into its golden age of popularity.

In 1906, however, the Pure Food and Drug Act was passed, prohibiting the interstate transportation of adulterated or misbranded food and drugs. In effect, the act brought about the decline of the patent medicine industry, because, henceforth, the proportions of cocaine, alcohol, opium, morphine, heroin, and a number of other substances in each preparation had to be indicated. And because of the mass media efforts to point out the negative effects of these ingredients, a number of the remedies lost their appeal—including those containing cocaine. Subsequently, cocaine use moved underground to the netherworlds of vice and crime, the jazz scene, and the bohemia of the avant-garde, where its major devotees included prostitutes, musicians, fortune-tellers, criminals, and members of minority groups. There it remained for decades, so much so that in 1939, the Treasury Department's Bureau of Narcotics concluded that "the use of cocaine in the illicit traffic continues to be so small as to be without significance" (Bureau of Narcotics, 1939, p. 14).

During the late 1960s and early 1970s, cocaine use began to move from the underground to mainstream society—to a great extent, the result of a series of decisions made at that time in Washington, D.C. First, the U.S. Senate and the federal drug-enforcement bureaucracy sponsored legislation that served to reduce the legal production of amphetamine-type drugs in the United States and to place strict controls on Quaaludes and other abused sedatives. Second and most important, the World Bank allocated funds for the construction of the Pan-American Highway through the Huallaga River valley in the high jungles of Peru. These two factors combined to usher in the cocaine era (Inciardi, 1992, p. 82).

The growing of coca leaves had always been popular on the slopes of the Peruvian Andes, but cultivation was for the most part limited for local consumption in tea or for chewing. Only relatively small amounts of the leaves were available for processing into cocaine. Travel throughout the rugged Andes terrain was difficult, and the coca leaves had to be carried out by mule pack. The World Bank's construction of a paved thoroughfare through the Huallaga valley opened up transportation routes for the shipping of coca, and the reduced availability of amphetamines and sedatives in the United States helped to provide a ready market for the new intoxicant. With the North Americans' increasing use of cocaine, South American growers and entrepreneurs responded by opening vast new areas for the cultivation of coca (Morales, 1989; Nicholl, 1985).

Cocaine in the 1980s and 1990s

Cocaine is often referred to as *coke, big C, lady, girl, snow, toot,* and *nose candy* (and, curiously, in Brazil as *Xuxa,* named after a popular television personality because of her white skin and blond hair). Regardless of these street names, the aura surrounding today's "coke" is quite different from that of Angelo Mariani's Vin Coca,

John Pemberton's French Wine Coca, or even Sigmund Freud's cocaine. Cocaine use in contemporary America is considered a major health problem, with estimates of the number of users ranging as high as 23 million (Weiss, Mirin, & Bartel, 1994).

Lured by its promise of intense and oftentimes orgasmic pleasure, millions of Americans use cocaine each year—a snort in each nostril, and the user is up and away for 20 minutes or so. Alert, witty, and with it—with no hangover, no lung cancer, and no holes in the arms or burned-out cells in the brain. The cocaine high is an immediate, intensely vivid, and sensation-enhancing experience. Moreover, it has the reputation for being a spectacular aphrodisiac: It is believed to create sexual desire, to heighten it, to increase sexual endurance, and to cure frigidity and impotence.

Given all these positives, no wonder cocaine became the all-American drug of the 1980s. And its use continues to permeate all levels of society. Yet, the pleasure and feelings of power that cocaine engenders make its use a problematic recreational pursuit. In the majority of cases, very small and occasional doses of cocaine are no more harmful than equally moderate doses of alcohol or marijuana and infinitely less so than heroin. But there is a side to cocaine that can be very destructive. The euphoric lift that comes from but a few brief snorts is short-lived and invariably followed by a letdown.

Because the body does not develop any significant tolerance to cocaine, and because physical dependence similar to that with heroin never develops, many cocaine users believe that the drug is non-addicting. Yet, this position is easily refuted, given the many chronic users who compulsively indulge in cocaine. Sidney Cohen of the Neuropsychiatric Institute at the Los Angeles School of Medicine, for example, suggests that the notion that cocaine does not produce addiction comes from the early professional literature, written at a time when the quantities of the drug used were smaller than those taken by contemporary users (Cohen, 1984). He adds that the high doses of cocaine currently used, combined with the frequency with which they are taken, produce a withdrawal syndrome characterized primarily by psychological depression. Others feel that what seems to be happening in these cases is only strong psychic dependence. Compulsive users seek the extreme mood elevation, elation, and grandiose feelings of heightened mental and physical prowess induced by the drug. When these begin to wane, a corresponding deep depression is felt, which is in such marked contrast to the users' previous states that they are strongly motivated to repeat the dose and restore their euphoria. Thus, when chronic users try to stop using cocaine, they are often plunged into a severe depression from which only the drug can arouse them.

In addition to the dependence potential, chronic cocaine use typically causes hyperstimulation, digestive disorders, nausea, loss of appetite, weight loss, tooth erosion, brain abscess, stroke, cardiac irregularities, occasional convulsions, and sometimes, paranoid psychoses and delusions of persecution (Fishel, Hamamoto, Barbul, Niji, & Efron, 1985; Gawin & Ellinwood, 1988; Grabowski, 1984). Moreover, repeated inhalation can result in erosions of the mucous membranes, including perforations of the nasal septum. A chronic runny nose is often a mark of the regular cocaine user (Rodriguez, 1989). Then, there are the effects of cocaine use during pregnancy, which are discussed at length in later chapters. These are the effects of snorting cocaine, the most common method of ingestion, but there are other ways of taking the drug, each of which can bring on an added spectrum of complications. One of these methods is *freebasing,* a phenomenon that has been known in the drug community for some two decades but moved into the mainstream of cocaine use during the 1980s. Cocaine hydrochloride has a high melting point and, thus, cannot be efficiently smoked. As a result, some users produce a change in the cocaine salt form to a base form. More specifically, freebase cocaine is actually a different chemical product from cocaine itself. In the process of preparing freebase, street cocaine, which is usually in the form of a hydrochloride salt, is treated with a liquid base (such as buffered ammonia) to remove the hydrochloric acid. The "free" cocaine (cocaine in the base state, free of the hydrochloric acid, and hence the name *freebase*) is then dissolved in a solvent such as ether, from which the purified cocaine is crystallized. These crystals, having a lower melting point, are then crushed and used in a special heated glass pipe. Smoking freebase cocaine provides a quicker and more potent rush or high and a far more powerful euphoric lift than regular cocaine and, as such, its use is that much more seductive. Moreover, the freebasing process involves the use of ether, a highly volatile petroleum product that has exploded in the face of many a user.

Cocaine has also been used as a sex aid, a practice that has brought both pleasurable and disastrous results. A sprinkle of cocaine on the clitoris or just below the head of the penis will anesthetize the tissues and retard a sexual climax. But with persistent stimulation, the drug will ultimately promote an explosive orgasm. However, the urethra (the tube inside the penis or the vulva through which urine is eliminated) is very sensitive to cocaine. At a minimum, the drug will dry out the urethral membranes, which must remain moist to function properly. At a maximum, because the absorption rate of cocaine through the walls of the urethra is quite rapid, overdoses have been known to happen (Macdonald, Waldorf, Reinarman, & Murphy, 1988).

As an aphrodisiac, cocaine is highly questionable. Research has found considerable differences in sexual responses to the same dosage level of cocaine, depending primarily on the setting of the use and the background experiences of the users. It is interesting that sexual response to cocaine is often different among men versus women. For men, cocaine typically helps to prevent premature ejaculation and at the same time permits prolonged intercourse before orgasm. Among women, achieving a climax under the influence of cocaine is often quite difficult. Research also demonstrates that chronic, heavy users of cocaine typically experience sexual dysfunction (Macdonald et al., 1988).

Among chronic users of cocaine, the practice of injecting the drug started to become more noticeable by the mid-1980s. This route of administration produces an extremely rapid onset of the drug's effects, usually within 15 to 20 seconds, along with a rather powerful high. It also produces the more debilitating effects of psychoses and paranoid delusions. A related phenomenon is the injection of cocaine in combination with another drug. Known as *speedballing,* the practice is not at all new. The classic speedball is a mixture of heroin and cocaine. It was referred to as such by the heroin-using community as early as the 1930s and as *whizbang* as far back as 1918 (Partridge, 1961, pp. 665, 770; Spears, 1981, p. 369; Wentworth & Flexner, 1975, p. 507). Whether the user's primary drug of choice is cocaine or heroin, the speedball intensifies the euphoric effect. Whether the pattern of use involves snorting, freebasing, shooting, speedballing, or smoking (discussed in the following section), the hazards of cocaine use can go well beyond those already noted. Some individuals, likely few in number, are hypersensitive to cocaine, and as little as 20 milligrams can be fatal. Because cocaine is a potent stimulant that rapidly increases the blood pressure, sudden death can also occur from only small amounts among users suffering from coronary artery disease or weak cerebral blood vessels. Cocaine is also a convulsant that can induce major seizures and cause fatalities if emergency treatment is not immediately at hand. Postcocaine depression, if intense, can lead to suicide. If the dose is large enough, cocaine can be toxic and result in an overdose. For the majority of users, this can occur with as little as 1 gram, taken intravenously. When injecting cocaine, furthermore, the user is also at high risk of exposure to infections that result from the use of unsterile needles— hepatitis and even HIV/AIDS.

And then there is crack, clearly the most seductive form of cocaine.

Crack Cocaine

Crack has been called the fast-food variety of cocaine. It is cheap, easy to conceal, it vaporizes with practically no odor, and the gratification is swift: an intense, almost sexual euphoria that lasts less than 5 minutes. Contrary to popular belief, crack is not a new substance, having been first reported in the literature during the early 1970s (*The Gourmet Cokebook*, 1972). At that time, however, knowledge of crack, known then as *base* or *rock,* seemed to be restricted to segments of cocaine's freebasing subculture. Crack is processed from cocaine hydrochloride by using ammonia or baking soda and water and heating it to remove the hydrochloride. The result is a pebble-sized crystalline form of cocaine base.

Contrary to another popular belief, crack is neither freebase cocaine nor purified cocaine. Part of the confusion about what crack actually is comes from the different ways that the word *freebase* is used in the drug community. Freebase (the substance) is a drug, a cocaine product converted to the base state from cocaine hydrochloride after adulterants have been chemically removed. Crack is converted to the base state without removing the adulterants. Freebasing (the act) means to inhale vapors of cocaine base, of which crack is but one form. Last, crack is not purified cocaine, because during its processing, the baking soda remains as a salt, thus reducing its homogeneity somewhat. Moreover, crack contains much of the filler and impurities found in the original cocaine hydrochloride, along with traces of baking soda and other residue.

As to the presence of crack in the drug communities of the early 1970s, it was available for only a short period of time before it was discarded by freebase-cocaine aficionados as an inferior product. Many of them referred to it as *garbage freebase* because of the many impurities it contained. The rediscovery of crack occurred early in the 1980s, and the drug was an immediate success, for a variety of reasons. First, it could be smoked rather than snorted. When cocaine is smoked, it is more rapidly absorbed and crosses the blood-brain barrier within 6 seconds. Hence, an almost instantaneous high.

Second, it was cheap. A gram of cocaine for snorting may cost $60 or more depending on its purity; the same gram can be transformed into anywhere from 5 to 30 "rocks." For the user, this meant that individual rocks could be purchased for as little as $2, $5 (nickel rocks), $10 (dime rocks), or $20. For the seller, $60 worth of cocaine hydrochloride (purchased wholesale for $30) could generate as much as $100 to $150 when sold as rocks. Third, it was easily hidden and transportable, and when hawked in small glass vials, it could be readily scrutinized by potential buyers.

The use of crack proliferated throughout the 1980s and into the 1990s. Subsequent to the initial media sensationalism, press coverage targeted the involvement of youths in crack distribution; the violence associated with struggles to control the crack marketplace in inner-city neighborhoods; and the child abuse, child neglect, and child abandonment by crack-addicted mothers (Revkin, 1989; Rosenbaum, 1987). Moreover, the production, sale, and use of crack, as well as prostitution and sex for drugs exchanges, became prominent features of the crack scene (Belenko, 1993; Inciardi, Lockwood, & Pottieger, 1993; Ratner, 1993; Williams, 1992).

Many crack users are uncertain as to what crack actually is. Some know it as cocaine that has been cooked into a hard, solid form, called a rock, or freebase. The preparation of crack is done in a variety of ways, all of which require baking soda, water, and an expander of some sort to increase its volume and weight and hence, the profits. Typical in this regard are such cocaine analogues as novocaine, lidocaine, and benzocaine, which will bind with the cocaine when cooked.

Crack is smoked in a variety of ways—typically, in either special glass pipes or makeshift smoking devices fabricated from beer or soda cans, jars, bottles, and other containers. Crack is also smoked with marijuana in cigarettes. Users typically smoke for as long as they have crack or the means to purchase it—money or sex, stolen goods, furniture, or other drugs. It is rare that smokers have but a single hit. More likely, they spend $50 to $500 during a so-called mission—a 3-day or 4-day binge, smoking almost constantly, 3 to 50 rocks per day. During these cycles, crack users rarely eat or sleep. And once crack is tried, for many users it is not long before it becomes a daily habit.

Crack smoking is often done in a crack house. The term *crack house* can mean a number of different things—a place to use crack, to sell it or to do both, or a place to manufacture and package crack. The location may be a house, an apartment, a small shack at the back of an empty lot, an abandoned building, or even the rusting hulk of an discarded automobile (see Ratner, 1993).

In addition to all of the problems associated with cocaine, there are additional complications with crack use. Smoking cocaine as opposed to snorting it results in more immediate and direct absorption of the drug, producing a quicker and more compelling high, greatly increasing the dependence potential. Moreover, there is increased risk of acute toxic reactions, including brain seizure, cardiac irregularities, respiratory paralysis, paranoid psychosis, and pulmonary dysfunction.

The tendency to binge on crack for days at a time, neglecting food, sleep, and basic hygiene, severely compromises physical health. As such, crack users appear emaciated most of the time. They lose interest in their physical appearance. Many have scabs on their faces, arms, and legs, the results of burns and picking on the skin (to remove bugs and other insects believed to be crawling under the skin). Crack users tend to have burned facial hair from carelessly lighting their smoking paraphernalia, they have burned lips and tongues from the hot stems of their pipes, and they seem to cough constantly. The tendency of both male and female crack users to engage in high frequency, unprotected sex with numerous anonymous partners increases their risk for any variety of sexually transmitted diseases, including AIDS. And too, there are the problems associated with crack-exposed infants.

Women, Drugs, and Drug-Abusing Women

Scientific research on drug abuse in the United States has but a short history, beginning just over a century ago (Terry & Pellens, 1928), and with the great majority of studies occurring only since the onset of the 1960s. Much of this work is concerned with either male alcoholism or male heroin addiction, which presents several difficulties for understanding cocaine use among women. First, research on cocaine users is quite limited, a situation understandably related to the only-recent appearance of cocaine in significant quantities in the U.S. drug scene. Second, and most notable, is the long tradition of ignoring gender as a drug-use variable. It is interesting in this regard that in 1975, a group of women at the Addiction Research Foundation questioned whether enough was known about women's substance abuse to justify attempting to publish an entire book on the subject (Kalant, 1980). Thus, intensive research on socially problematic drug use among women is only as old as the cocaine problem itself. Although this field of study has made enormous strides in the past two decades, its limited history continues to restrict the amount of information available to understand and deal with the issues associated with women and cocaine. Furthermore, the inclination to ignore women in drug research persists. This makes a brief look at the history of research on women's drug problems a useful starting point for examining the more focused topic of cocaine-exposed infants.

Studies of Women and Drugs

Most of the research on women and drug use undertaken prior to the early 1970s involved clinical analyses of female heroin addicts and alcoholics, often labeling them as self-destructive, unstable, sexually maladjusted, insecure, and socially immature (see Burt, Glynn, & Sowder, 1979; Colten, 1979). As Dr. Barbara G. Lex (1991) of the Harvard Medical School points out in the specific case of alcohol, the determination that female substance abusers were suffering from severe psychological maladies came at a time when many researchers were suggesting that gender was irrelevant to studies of chemical dependence. Many in the field of drug research still assumed that substance abuse was essentially a male problem because sociocultural factors protected women from involvement in highly deviant behavior.

By the 1970s, drug problems among women began to gain importance as a subject for research. The eruption of drug use among adolescents and young adults in the 1960s provoked a major change in how illicit drug use was viewed. The psychiatric domain of drug abuse gave way to peer group and subcultural explanations of substance abuse. Ethnographic studies of male heroin users, which showed them to be alert, resourceful, purposive hustlers engaged in numerous activities for the sake of securing heroin and avoiding arrest, contrasted sharply with the view that they were psychologically deficient (see Agar, 1973; Feldman, 1968; Preble & Casey, 1969; Sutter, 1966). These studies of male street culture became the forerunners of later research on female heroin users.

Increasing rates of substance abuse also spurred the first large-scale epidemiologic studies of illicit drug use. And in fact, these surveys indicated that many adolescents and young adults in the general population were using illegal drugs. Rates of marijuana use among female students were found to be surprisingly high, and most rates of increase for illicit drug use by young women surpassed those for young men in the 1967 to 1972 period (Cisin, Miller, & Harrell, 1978).

Another important factor that led to in-depth drug studies of women was the heroin epidemics of the 1960s. Heroin use accounted for much of the general increase in illicit drug use during this time, with a major epidemic peaking in the late 1960s in large metropolitan areas (Greene, 1974; Hunt & Chambers, 1976). Women's rates of heroin use did in fact rise more quickly than did those for males, as indicated by national arrest rates for narcotic offenses and gender distributions of addicts appearing for treatment (Cuskey, Richardson, & Berger, 1979; Nurco, Wegner, Baum, & Makotsky, 1979; Prather & Fidell, 1978; Ramer, Smith, & Gay, 1972). By the mid-1970s, women composed about one quarter of the heroin addicts entering treatment. As this represented a 33% increase from figures reported just 10 years earlier, it became increasingly apparent to some clinicians that women's treatment needs would have to be given more attention.

The 1975 to 1985 time period also saw several other new kinds of research on women and substance abuse. In-depth interviews were conducted on a large scale with street-active female heroin users (users who were not in treatment or prison), and a notable ethnography of women heroin users and their lives on the street was initiated by Marsha Rosenbaum of the Institute for Scientific Analysis in San Francisco (Rosenbaum, 1981).

As a consequence of the new research attention to women, significant progress was made in understanding the motivations for women's drug and alcohol involvement, gender differences in substance abuse patterns, and contrasts between women involved in alternative types or levels of substance abuse and women from similar backgrounds who were not drug involved. At the same time, however, traditional research limitations have continued. Pregnancy and psychopathology often remain primary interests for studies of women's drug use, and reports continue to appear with all-male samples or, more commonly, analyses that ignore gender (see Lex, 1991).

Based in part on the work of early researchers, those in the field of drug abuse today recognize that multidimensional analyses and attention to linkages between drug use and other socially problematic behaviors are crucial components of useful research (for example, see Reed, 1991). However, examinations of existing single-drug research from a comparative perspective can also be useful. This body of research indicates that women's experiences with substance abuse are strikingly similar, regardless of the drug's legal status or psychopharmacological properties. Whether the drug of choice is alcohol, heroin, or cocaine, both inner-city and middle-class women are likely to report similar initial drug-use situations and have similar motives for taking drugs. In addition, many experience the same kinds of problems as they increase their drug use. Differential experiences that are introduced by the use of so-called harder street drugs (such as crack) may include additional life problems that are encountered by these users. Within this context, it is helpful to recognize the psychological, social, and cultural experience of stig-matization associated with women's drug abuse. The stigma associ-ated with drug abuse by a woman is both the most consistent and most consequential similarity in the experiences of drug-involved women. Such behavior violates female role expectations so seriously that it can result in social isolation, cultural denigration, and feelings of shame that help to perpetuate the very behavior at issue.

With what is known about the consequences of women's chemical dependency, what motivates and maintains their drug use? Among both male and female adolescents, drug-use initiation often occurs out of curiosity and the desire to experiment with new behaviors. However, motivation for continued use is different for men and women. Females are much less likely than males to use illegal drugs for thrills or pleasure or to use alcohol and drugs in response to peer pressure. Instead, women are more likely to use any and all drug types for self-medication—that is, as a coping mechanism for dealing with situational factors, life events, or general psychological distress (Griffin, Weiss, Mirin, & Lange, 1989; Hser, Anglin, & Booth, 1987; Novacek, Raskin, & Hogan, 1991; Reed, 1991; Suffet & Brotman, 1976). Depression is a particularly common problem among chemically dependent women, and unlike men, women's depression likely occurs before, rather than after, the development of a drug problem (see Blume, 1990). The importance of such factors is corroborated by the repeated finding that counseling to foster self-esteem and a sense of personal competence are critical elements in successful treatment of drug dependence in women.

Still other problems motivating self-medication may stem from traumas of personal history, particularly rape, incest, and other sex-ual abuse. Such histories are much more usual among women than men and have been found to be extremely common among women with drug problems (Reed, 1991; Stevens, Arbiter, & Glider, 1989; Vandor, Juliana, & Leone, 1991; Wilsnack, 1984). A recent study of 572 women in substance-abuse treatment also demonstrated that drug abuse is increasingly common in the histories of younger women compared with earlier cohorts. Although they were only slightly more likely to experience childhood sexual abuse, younger women were more often involved with men who abused them both sexually and physically (Harrison, 1989).

Women are also subject to greater economic pressures, because they are less likely than men to have adequate job income and, more often than not, are responsible for their children's support. In fact, most women entering drug treatment are described as having inadequate levels of education and job training and extremely high rates of unemployment (Inciardi et al., 1993).

Regardless of the motivating factors, women who establish a pattern of heavy drug use undergo many analogous experiences. One experience that is not unique to women is that any problem drug use today tends to be multiple drug use. Alcohol and prescription drug combinations appear particularly often among women, whereas heroin users commonly prefer speedballs (typically, a combination of heroin and cocaine) plus marijuana and pills. Cocaine users often use considerable amounts of some kind of depressant, typically alcohol, and the great majority also use marijuana. The use of multiple drugs is problematic because it complicates and exacerbates the user's addiction pattern and the effect of drugs on the user's body, both of which make treatment efforts all the more difficult.

Another common problem for chemically dependent men and women is impaired sexual functioning. This includes physiological damage, disruption of reproductive functioning, and diminished sexual interest. The latter is of particular interest in that many recreational drugs—including alcohol, marijuana, inhalants, heroin, and cocaine (as mentioned earlier in this chapter)—have been reputed to be aphrodisiacs. Although the aphrodisiac claim may have some psychopharmacological basis when used in moderation, excessive use is almost always associated with impaired functioning and a devotion to drug use that permits little interest in any other activity (Macdonald et al., 1988). Impaired sexual functioning for chemically dependent women may also pertain to their male partners' drug-related sexual dysfunctions, which include impotence and lack of sexual interest.

A chemical dependency problem necessarily unique to women is complications in pregnancy and childbirth. Alcohol, cocaine, heroin, marijuana, PCP, and prescription sedatives and tranquilizers have all been implicated in studies of maternal drug use and fetal harm. As is noted in later chapters, because these drugs are able to cross the placental barrier to affect the fetus, children born to chemically dependent women may be subject to problems that increase the risk of both neonatal mortality and significant long-term developmental disabilities.

The subject of pregnancy complications, fetal damage, and child impairment is one that illustrates particularly well the gaps in existing knowledge about both women's drug use and linkages between substance abuse and other socially problematic behaviors. That is, although many of the physiological effects discussed have been seen in animal studies, indicating a direct drug effect, others have not. One reason is the previously mentioned lack of female-centered drug-abuse research studies. An additional consideration is that drug involvement is almost never a woman's sole life problem, and it can be an arduous task to separate the effects of drug use from those of other difficulties.[1] In the case of pregnancy and childbirth, especially pertinent complications often seen among drug users include poverty, sexually transmitted diseases, cigarette smoking, poor nutritional status and general health, and little or no prenatal care. Thus, the effects of drug use, specifically cocaine, are difficult to identify for at least three reasons: (a) the drug is so rapidly metabolized that urine tests even a few hours after last use may not show its presence, (b) the likelihood that cocaine users also use multiple other drugs, and (c) the markedly high probability that pregnant cocaine users will receive little or no prenatal care.

In addition to fetal health concerns, substance abuse of all types has a general deleterious effect on the health of the user, and many such problems appear to be more significant for women than men (see Lex, 1991). Part of the explanation is simple physiology: Compared to men, women have a smaller average body weight, less body water per pound, and more body fat per pound. Thus, a water-soluble substance, such as alcohol or cocaine, will result in higher blood or plasma drug levels for women even if dosage and body size are constant. For fat-soluble drugs, such as marijuana and minor tranquilizers, fatty tissue will store and gradually release the drug into a woman's system over a longer period of time than will occur for a man (see Blume, 1990; Lex, 1991). Furthermore, the liver is the organ that breaks down poisons—such as alcohol and other drugs—taken into the body, and the female sex hormone estrogen apparently has an adverse effect on liver functioning. At high levels of drug intake, women thus develop physiological problems after a shorter period of years. Female alcoholics have a more rapid development of cardiovascular, gastrointestinal, and liver diseases. And, whereas mortality rates for male alcoholics are 2 or 3 times higher than those for men of similar ages in the general population, women alcoholics suffer 2.7 to 7 times as many deaths (Lex, 1991). Similarly, drug dependence itself appears to occur more rapidly among women, a finding reported for alcohol, heroin, and cocaine.

Despite the significant health consequences of substance abuse for women, placement in appropriate treatment settings has been difficult. Even when the need for treatment is recognized, women seeking help are likely to enter a program that does not meet their needs because it was originally designed for men. An often encountered problem in treatment settings is the type of therapy administered. Successful group therapy for chemically dependent men, for example, often involves confrontations by peers to help them recognize and admit their underlying problems. In contrast, women tend to react negatively to confrontational techniques and instead, benefit from intensive mutual support from peers. Women also require a wider range of ancillary services for successful treatment—notably, a broader range of medical and psychological assistance, help with child care (possibly to even enter treatment in the first place), and services aimed at reducing the extreme isolation typical of women drug users, such as mutual support groups and family therapy (see Beckman & Amaro, 1984; Stevens et al., 1989). Because these services require additional financing, they are not as common as one might wish. Even the language traditionally used by therapists and support groups, such as Alcoholics Anonymous, Cocaine Anonymous, and Narcotics Anonymous, can be a problem for women. A male psychiatrist with extensive experience treating cocaine users has stated,

> I feel I'm reasonably sensitive to the times we live in, and I know that women tend to feel more disempowered and disenfranchised. But once when I told a woman she was not surrendering to her healing process, she correctly admonished me that women have been advised all of their lives to stay humble and surrender, and it's gotten them nothing but more victimization and subjugation. (see Greenleaf, 1989, pp. 24-25)

Although great progress has been made over the past 15 years in designing treatment programs more suitable for women, male-oriented treatment facilities remain a problem shared by chemically dependent women regardless of the drugs they use.

Nonetheless, women appear to be involved in chemical dependency for shorter durations than men. This situation has been documented among heavy users of alcohol in the general population, as well as for alcohol, heroin, and cocaine users prior to treatment entry (Anglin, Hser, & Booth, 1987; Beckman & Amaro, 1984). One mitigating factor may be that women are often motivated to discontinue drug use out of concern for their children, a consideration that is oftentimes less compelling for men. Ironically, children can also be a significant barrier to women's treatment entry, because many programs continue to ignore the child care needs of their female clients. Pregnancy can likewise motivate a woman to seek treatment, but there continues to be a shortage of drug treatment programs that will accept pregnant women. The efforts to have pregnant addicts prosecuted for child abuse or delivering drugs in utero has necessarily served to push more women away from treatment (see Chapter 4).

Postscript

Cocaine has been portrayed in both the scientific and popular literature as a drug with particular appeal to women. The motivations suggested cover a broad range of interests:

1. Cocaine imparts a feeling of self-confidence and empowerment—and women are particularly prone to impaired self-esteem and feelings of powerlessness. The appeal of cocaine may be especially strong for women with a childhood history of abuse and neglect, which describes a larger percentage of chemically dependent females than of their male counterparts.

2. Cocaine, as a central nervous system stimulant, makes users feel energetic, competent, productive, and enthusiastic—and women are particularly subject to depression. Furthermore, women's dual workforce and home obligations mean that they are especially likely to have both physically and emotionally exhausting daily schedules.

3. Cocaine increases libido, at least for occasional to moderate use, which women may find helpful given modern expectations of women's so-called sexual liberation, in the face of continuing ambivalent socialization for women about the permissibility of sexual expression.

4. Cocaine suppresses interest in food, and women are particularly likely to be concerned about body size and on diets. Weight loss is generally

only a discovered side effect rather than an initial reason for use, but women are likely to see it as a positive reason to continue using cocaine.

5. Snorting cocaine and smoking crack permit self-administration of a powerful drug without resorting to needle use, a drug-use technique that women are more reluctant than men to initiate.

6. Cocaine use averts some incapacitating side effects of depressants, which may put female users at increased risk for victimization, especially sexual assault.

This list is impressively varied, but it has several flaws in logic. Given the literature on women and drugs just reviewed, perhaps the most obvious flaw is that none of the cited appeals is unique to cocaine. Stimulant effects, including self-confidence, energy, weight loss, and a high without drowsiness, are available with prescription drugs. Also, many different drugs relieve depression and anxiety (including sexual anxiety), and most do not involve needle use.

A second logical flaw is that, on the face of it, cocaine seems obviously more appealing to men than women because its primary effect is to make the user feel powerful, competent, in total command—certainly a more stereotypically male than female concern. Third and relatedly, one can easily argue that the drug effects that should appeal to women more than any other are those of heroin. As one of Marsha Rosenbaum's informants told her, "It's just a good feeling. At that particular time, shit, you don't have a problem in the world. Nothin'. At the time you are loaded, nothing bothers you" (Rosenbaum, 1981, p. 44).

So why has no one argued that heroin is the perfect trap for women? Most likely, because it is too exclusively associated with street life to be a meaningful option to most women. Cocaine, on the other hand, can be given such a label because it also has associations with Hollywood, Wall Street, and the lives of the rich and famous. But such lifestyles bear no more relationship to the lives of average U.S. women than do the netherworlds of street addicts. This suggests another flaw in the logic of seeing cocaine as the ultimately attractive drug for women—it isn't any more real to most women than is heroin.

Patricia G. Erickson and Glenn F. Murray of the Addiction Research Foundation also disagree with the claim of cocaine's special appeal to women, calling it greatly overstated because (a) more males than females use cocaine, (b) there is no evidence that female rates of use are growing faster than those for males, and (c) there is likewise no evidence that (among typical users not in treatment or jail) women are more susceptible to cocaine's effects (Erickson & Murray, 1989, p. 150). These researchers conclude that the primary reason for the greater publicity given to women's cocaine involvement is that a sexual double standard is being applied. Women's cocaine use is seen as more alarming than men's because it is connected to both old ideas about women's drug use being a source of sexual corruption and newer ideas about women's workforce participation leading to new pressures and temptations for women because they are taking on male role characteristics. In short, women who use cocaine "are subject to considerably more negative stereotyping and social repercussions than are men who engage in the same behavior" (Erickson & Murray, 1989, p. 150).

With respect to the extent to which women use cocaine and crack, many different mechanisms have been used to classify cocaine users into different groups. Some classifications have been based on frequency and amount of use, whereas others have focused on motivations, routes of administration, or contexts of use (see Stone, Fromme, & Kogan, 1984). Perhaps the most practical way of differentiating types of cocaine users is the simple fourfold classification of experimenters, social-recreational users, involved users, and dysfunctional abusers—a general classification that has been widely applied in the drug field for quite some time.

The experimenters are by far the largest group of cocaine users. They most frequently try cocaine a time or two in a social setting, but the drug does not play a significant role in their lives. They use cocaine experimentally because their social group relates the drug's effects as being pleasurable. Experimenters do not seek out cocaine but may use it when someone presents it to them in an appropriate setting. In this situation, they may use the drug (typically, by snorting it) once or twice because it does something *to* them.

Social-recreational users differ from experimenters primarily in terms of frequency and continuity of consumption. For example, they may use cocaine when they are at a party and someone presents the opportunity. Cocaine still does not play a significant role in these users' lives. They still do not actively seek out the drug but use it only because it does something *to* them—it makes them feel good.

For involved users, a major transition has taken place since the social-recreational use phase. As users become involved with cocaine, they also become drug seekers, and cocaine becomes significant to their lives. Although they are still quite able to function—in school, on the job, or as a parent or spouse—their proficiency in

many areas begins to decline markedly. Personal and social functioning tends to be inversely related to the amount of time involved users
spend with cocaine. They still have control over their behavior, but
their use of the drug occurs with increasing frequency for some
adaptive reason; cocaine does something *for* them.

Involved cocaine users are of many types. Some use the drug to
deal with an unbearable work situation, indulging in controlled
amounts several times a day. Others use cocaine to enhance performance or bolster their self-esteem. And still a third group regularly
uses cocaine to deal with stress, anxiety, nagging boredom, or
hopelessness.

The dysfunctional abusers are those who have become known as
the *cokeheads, cokeaholics, cocaine addicts, crack whores.* For them,
cocaine has become the significant part of their lives. They are
personally and socially dysfunctional and spend all of their time in
cocaine seeking, cocaine taking, and other related activities. Moreover, they no longer have control over their cocaine use.

Because patterns of cocaine use transcend gender barriers,
women cocaine users can be of all four types—experimenters, social-
recreational users, involved users, and dysfunctional abusers.

Note

1. This issue is examined at length in Chapter 3.

2. "Cocaine Babies"

In 1987, Dr. Ira J. Chasnoff of Northwestern University Medical School in Chicago reported that between .4% and 27% of pregnant women seen in hospitals across the United States were drug abusers. By multiplying the 11% average against live births in the United States in 1987 (3,809,394), Chasnoff estimated that 375,000 infants were drug exposed each year (Besharov, 1990). Other researchers believed that his estimate was too high, particularly for cocaine exposure. For example, a survey conducted by the National Institute on Drug Abuse (NIDA) in 1990 indicated that approximately 4.5% of pregnant women between the ages of 12 and 34 had used cocaine during pregnancy. This would have placed the number of exposed infants at around 158,400 (Gomby & Shiono, 1991).[1]

Early research on the effects of prenatal substance abuse in the mid-1980s characterized cocaine-exposed children as moody, often inconsolable, less socially interactive, and less able to bond than other children (Fackelmann, 1991; Lester et al., 1991; Rothman, 1991). Many researchers also found drug-exposed children to be less attentive and less able to focus on specific tasks than nonexposed children (Chasnoff, Burns, Schnoll, & Burns, 1985; Chasnoff, Griffith, MacGregor, Dirkes, & Burns, 1989; Colen, 1990; Pinkney, 1989;

Rothman, 1991). Other harmful effects attributed to prenatal cocaine exposure included high rates of placental abruption (detach-
ment of the placenta from the uterine wall), *placenta previa* (location
of the placenta in front of the birth canal), growth retardation in
utero (in the uterus), sudden infant death syndrome (SIDS), withdrawal symptoms, cerebral infarctions (death of brain tissue due to
loss of blood supply), low birth weight, physical malformations,
microcephaly (small head circumference), and genitourinary tract
malformations.[2] Disturbances of feeding, sleep, and vision were also
reported (Bingol, Fuchs, Diaz, Stone, & Gromisch, 1987; Chasnoff,
Chisum, & Kaplan, 1988; Chasnoff & Griffith, 1989; Chasnoff,
Schnell, & Burns, 1986; Kim, Chicola, Noble, & Yoon, 1989). Many
studies frequently characterized these effects as irreversible and
suggested that no amount of special attention or educational programs would ever be able to turn these cocaine-exposed infants into
well-functioning or adjusted children (Colen, 1990; Public Health
Foundation, 1990). For example, the following account of a white,
middle-class cocaine user whose newborn son evidenced problems
likely related to her drug use appeared in the journal *Childbirth
Educator* in 1986:

> Mrs. Marshall (a pseudonym) used cocaine during the first five weeks of
> her pregnancy and then snorted five grams of cocaine over three days in
> the last week of her pregnancy. She noticed that her baby became
> extremely active during the first two days she used the drug; on the third
> day she used a large dose of cocaine and the baby stopped moving. Three
> hours after the last dose her contractions began. When she was admitted
> to the hospital, she was disoriented and her speech was slurred. Her heart
> rate was 120 beats per minute (bpm); that of the fetus was 180 to 200
> bpm.
>   A baby boy was born 15 hours after she last used cocaine. He was
> limp, and his heart rate had dropped to 80 bpm. He was given oxygen
> briefly and markedly improved. He appeared normal except for mildly
> decreased muscle tone of the right arm and a fast heart rate of 180 bpm.
> When the baby was about 16 hours old, he stopped breathing and turned
> blue several times. Transferred to the high-risk nursery, he had several
> seizures on his right side and decreased muscle tone in his right arm,
> shoulder, and hip. He was given medication to control his seizures. His
> heart rate was intermittently high, and his blood pressure was also raised.
> An X ray of his brain performed when he was 24 hours old revealed that
> he had had a stroke. The stroke may have been caused either by his high
> blood pressure before and after birth and a subsequent cerebral hemorrhage

or by decreased blood flow to the brain caused by his low blood pressure and heart rate at birth. (Chasnoff, 1986/1987)

Cocaine (and Crack) Babies in the Media

Such dramatic findings sparked a wave of media reports lamenting the fate of a new generation of so-called "crack babies." Numerous media stories documented the epidemic numbers of cocaine-addicted infants being born in large, urban hospitals across the United States (Kerr, 1986; McNamara, 1989). More often than not, the media publicized case studies of a few children who had been profoundly affected by prenatal exposure to multiple drugs, not exclusively cocaine. However, headlines that read "The Crack Children," "Crack Babies Born to Life of Suffering," "A Desperate Crack Legacy," and "Crack in the Cradle" focused much of the public's attention on the dangers of cocaine and created the image that crack babies were severely damaged human beings (Hopkins, 1990; Kantrowitz & Wingert, 1990; Langone, 1988; Stone, 1989). Take, for example, the following excerpts from a story that appeared in the *New York Times* in 1989:

Babies born to mothers using crack have serious difficulty relating to their world, making friends, playing like normal children, and feeling love for their mother or primary caretakers. Prenatal exposure to illegal drugs, particularly powdered cocaine and crack, seems to be "interfering with the central core of what it is to be human," said Coryl Jones, a research psychologist at the National Institute on Drug Abuse. New research indicates that most babies exposed to illegal drugs appear to be able to develop normal, if low-range intelligence, despite their subnormal emotional development. But the studies suggest that children of addicted mothers may be unable to develop into adults with basic employment skills and unable to form close human relationships. (Blakeslee, 1989)

A similarly disturbing story appeared in *Newsweek* a few months later:

The problems of crack children are long-term and far more difficult to solve. Educators are frustrated and bewildered by their behavior. "They operate only on an instinctual level, something has been left out," says Geynille Agee of her students. . . . Dr. Judy Howard of the UCLA School of Medicine, who has studied hundreds of crack children, says that crack babies are extremely irritable, very lethargic, hyperactive, and may have trouble relating to other people. As part of her research Dr. Howard compared crack preemies with non-crack preemies. Even at the age of 18 months, the crack kids would hit or throw their toys. "The kids have an impairment that makes them disorganized in everything they do," she says. Dr. Howard says it's as if the part of the brain that "makes us human beings, capable of discussion or reflection," has been "wiped out." (Kantrowitz & Wingert, 1990, pp. 62-63)

Accounts of behavioral disturbances among cocaine-exposed children were particularly commonplace. As frightening reports from weary, disconcerted family members and teachers grew more frequent, public concern over this so-called lost generation increased. Consider the following excerpts, which ran in newspapers and magazines across the country. In the *Miami Herald,*

The tiny angelic looking boy is only 4 but he has long had a reputation around his day care center. For tantrums. He would hurl himself on the floor and bang his head against the concrete. The boy is a cocaine child—his fragile system damaged by the drug while he was still in the womb. . . . "They're like little Jekylls and Hydes" said a Fort Lauderdale school principal, "all of a sudden, something will set them off. They start throwing tantrums. They start yelling. They can't control their emotions." (Marks, 1990, p. A1)

In the *Wall Street Journal,*

One slim six year old boy sits on the floor with his classmates happily singing an alphabet song. Two years ago, he used to throw hour long tantrums. He would build a tower of blocks, then shout that it was on fire and knock it down. Last year, while classmates watched the space shuttle blast off on television, he banged on his desk and cried. Extremes of behavior are common, from apathy to aggression, passivity to hyperactivity, indiscriminate trust to extreme suspicion. Teachers also see more subtle signs of the children's drug exposure and fragmented lives. A girl demands to be left alone, bumps into walls, or stares blankly into space. A boy screams and throws himself on the floor because he wants to be picked up but can't express himself. (Trost, 1989, p. A1)

In the *New York Times,*

One couple who adopted a child said in an interview that they were unaware that they were rearing a baby exposed to drugs in the womb.

He was jittery and wailed nonstop, he wouldn't react to sound. He seemed physically stiff. When he was 15 months old, he suffered grand mal epileptic seizures. He wouldn't make eye contact. He didn't want to be held. The boy is now 3, and is profoundly hyperactive and subject to intense rage. (Blakeslee, 1990, p. A1)

And in the *Washington Post,*

The kindergartners spill into their elementary school each morning bubbling with enthusiasm, but for some enthusiasm is not enough. . . . One of the students is so antsy that on some days [the teacher] helps him hold his pencil. The student can't concentrate for more than a few minutes at a time. The student also has problems gauging spatial relationships. He attempts to sit down at his seat and misses his chair altogether. The child also exhibits a seeming inability to control his emotions so that mild frustration rapidly ascends to temper tantrums and abusive behavior. (Norris, 1991, p. A1)

Portrayals of cocaine-exposed infants as children out of control, prone to hyperactivity, overstimulation, distractibility, seizures, fits of rage, and violent behavior certainly hampered efforts at finding caretakers for these children in need. By the late 1980s, many jurisdictions required physician reporting of drug use in pregnancy or positive drug tests from infants. Infants who test positive for cocaine are automatically kept in the hospital and because they are often born prematurely, they frequently require long hospital stays until they are declared medically fit to leave. Many times, however, even when the children become eligible to leave, the mother may either be unavailable or deemed unfit to care for them. The long search for adequate foster care then begins, giving rise to large numbers of so-called boarder babies in many urban hospitals (McNamara, 1989; Thornton, 1988/1989).[3]

Reports that suggested that cocaine-damaged children would face insurmountable educational and social obstacles that may doom them to failure in the future (Chira, 1990; Toufexis, 1991) and the media's tendency to cite studies with detrimental findings of cocaine exposure created something of a self-fulfilling prophecy (Greider, 1995). Children labeled as crack babies have been characterized as having little potential for successful outcomes, and as such, prospective adoptive parents have been unwilling to care for these kids, and schoolteachers have been prepared for the worst. Too often, the media's stereotypic portrayal of crack babies has obscured the fact that most children who are exposed to cocaine in utero are also exposed to other substances (Gonzalez & Campbell, 1994; Griffith, Azuma, & Chasnoff, 1994). Cocaine-using women are much more likely than nonusers to smoke cigarettes and use alcohol during pregnancy (Shiono et al., 1995). In fact, researchers estimate that the number of children exposed to alcohol in utero is almost 10 times greater than the number exposed to cocaine, affecting approximately 73% of all pregnancies (Scherling, 1994).

Indeed, NIDA (1994) has suggested that predictions of a so-called lost generation of cocaine-exposed children were overstated. NIDA has reported that approximately one half of all infants born to drug-using mothers have no drug-related health effects and has suggested that previous estimates of epidemic numbers of cocaine-affected infants resulted from the lack of representative samples and reliable data in early studies. In fact, many early research studies of prenatal cocaine exposure suffered from a variety of methodological flaws that may call their findings into question. For example, the initial reports that suggested that cocaine use caused a dramatic increase in the likelihood of SIDS were based on very small, non-representative samples (NIDA, 1989; Ward et al., 1989), making the generalizability of the findings questionable (Greider, 1995; Shiono et al., 1995).

Although one would like to think that members of the medical and research community always act in good faith while conducting their research and ensure that their studies are free from personal agendas, this may not always be the case. For example, in a 1989 issue of the prestigious British medical journal *The Lancet,* a report indicated that abstracts on the impact of cocaine use were more likely to be accepted for presentation at the annual meeting of the Society for Pediatric Research if the study found adverse effects of cocaine. Because studies that found minimal or no effects of cocaine were less likely to be approved, the bulk of the presentations demonstrated overwhelmingly that cocaine use was unduly harmful to both the mother and her fetus. Further examination found that in general, the rejected studies had better methodologies (they took into account more of the confounding variables, used larger sample sizes) than those that were accepted (Koren et al., 1989).

Moreover, several of the early and most well-publicized studies conducted on prenatal cocaine exposure by Dr. Ira Chasnoff and his colleagues have come under scrutiny in the past several years due to a number of troubling research design issues that may have tarnished some of their conclusions. For example, in 1985, Dr. Chasnoff published his initial report on the use of cocaine during pregnancy in the widely circulated and highly prominent *New England Journal of Medicine* (Chasnoff et al., 1985). Chasnoff and his colleagues conducted a study of 23 cocaine-using, pregnant women enrolled in a prenatal addiction project between January 1983 and September 1984. The 23 women were divided into two groups: 12 women using cocaine alone and 11 women using heroin in combination with cocaine. Two matched control groups included 15 women who were drug-free during pregnancy and 15 former heroin addicts who were in a methadone maintenance program throughout their pregnancies. All groups were said to be similar in maternal age, number of pregnancies, socioeconomic status, and degree of alcohol, marijuana, and tobacco use. The 53 infants born to these women were given thorough medical, neural, and behavioral assessments. Although no significant differences were found in gestational age (the length of time from conception to birth, as calculated from the first day of the last normal menstrual period), birth weight, length, or head circumference in any of the groups, one infant born to a cocaine-using woman was diagnosed with prune-belly syndrome, a congenital defect in which one or more layers of abdominal muscles are absent. Furthermore, the cocaine-using women in this study were said to have had a history of spontaneous abortion that was significantly higher than that of the heroin-using or drug-free women. In terms of behavior, the authors presented data that showed that infants exposed only to cocaine in utero suffered from decreased response to external stimuli.

The conclusions drawn from these data appear to be problematic for several reasons. In addition to questions raised by the very small and perhaps nonrepresentative sample, many of the researchers' summations were not supported by the data. Specifically, the authors' asserted that "it is possible to infer from these data that infants exposed to cocaine are at risk for a higher rate of congenital malformations and perinatal mortality" (Chasnoff et al., 1985, p. 669).

As mentioned earlier, however, the presence of a single infant born with prune-belly syndrome was the only malformation reported in the study, and statistical tests for association between cocaine use and congenital abnormalities were noticeably absent. The authors' reference to increased perinatal mortality among cocaine-using women may also be called into question. All of the women in the study delivered live infants, with no differences in gestational age between groups. The allusion to higher perinatal mortality among cocaine-using women was based on retrospective, self-reported drug use and pregnancy data collected on study participants. Although the authors acknowledged that temporal relations between specific episodes of drug use and spontaneous abortion could not be determined, they nevertheless concluded that "there had been a significantly increased rate of spontaneous abortion in previous pregnancies among the cocaine-using women" (Chasnoff et al., 1985, p. 667). In light of a number of issues surrounding the validity of self-report cocaine use (see Mieczkowski, 1990) and problems with patient recall, it is noteworthy that no corroboration of pregnancy history was obtained from the women's medical records.

Additional difficulties were noted in the inferences drawn from the analysis of these historical data. In the Chasnoff et al. (1985) study, cocaine-using women were defined as those who were using cocaine at the time of conception *in the current pregnancy*. The women's *current* group assignments (cocaine only, cocaine and heroin, methadone, drug free) were related to the occurrence of spontaneous abortion *in previous pregnancies*, although it was not clear whether the effects of *prior* cocaine use were associated with a higher rate of miscarriage. Based on these retrospective reports, the authors inferred a causal relationship that was obviously overstated: "[The] increased rate of spontaneous abortion found in cocaine-using women . . . is consistent with the pharmacologic actions of cocaine" (p. 668).

Discrepancies in behavioral data reports are also observable in this study. For example, scores on the Brazelton Neonatal Behavioral Assessment Scale, which was administered to each infant, revealed that cocaine-exposed infants showed poorer responses to environmental stimuli and that "infants exposed to methadone had significantly worse scores in the interactive cluster than did control infants" (Chasnoff et al., 1985, p. 668). However, in their concluding remarks, the authors presented the contradictory statement that it was not the methadone-using women but the cocaine-using women who had infants with the worst scores in the interactive cluster (Chasnoff et al., 1985, p. 669).

Even more serious, however, was the failure of early prenatal cocaine studies to disentangle the effects of cocaine exposure from exposure to alcohol, tobacco, other drugs, and other biological and environmental factors (Scherling, 1994; Shiono et al., 1995). One 1989 study on the effects of prenatal cocaine exposure illustrates this tendency to attribute negative health consequences to cocaine use despite the presence of other substance use (see Chasnoff et al., 1989). Briefly, infants born to two groups of women who had used cocaine during pregnancy, either continuously or exclusively in the first trimester, were medically evaluated and compared with the infants of a drug-free control group. Reported use of marijuana and alcohol was said to be similar among the cocaine-using sets, whereas the drug-free controls related no use of these substances. Based on medical and behavioral assessments, the researchers reported the following:

- Infants born to women who used cocaine throughout pregnancy had a lower mean weight, length, and head circumference at birth compared with the drug-free infants.
- The cocaine-exposed infants demonstrated significant impairment in the areas of orientation, motor ability, state regulation, and reflexes compared with the drug-free infants.

Building on these findings, Chasnoff et al. (1989) concluded that cocaine was responsible for decreases in intrauterine growth and that

Exposure to *cocaine* [italics added] in the prenatal period leads to significant impairment in neonatal neurobehavioral capabilities. This study further indicates that the neurobehavioral response deficiencies occur in the cocaine-exposed infant whether the mother stops cocaine use in the first trimester or uses cocaine throughout the pregnancy. (p. 1744)

Such sweeping inferences did not account for the interactive effects of cocaine when used in combination with other substances, and no attempt was made to isolate the consequences of cocaine, marijuana, and alcohol use. The use of inappropriate controls, who had no exposure to either alcohol or marijuana, made establishing meaningful linkages between cocaine use and its purported effects virtually an impossible task.

Multiple Drug Exposure

Whereas upwards of 50,000 cocaine-exposed infants are born in the United States each year, cocaine alone is rarely used by the mothers. Women who use cocaine while pregnant are also much more likely than other women to use alcohol, cigarettes, and other illegal drugs (Rosecan & Gross, 1986; Van Dyke & Fox, 1990), necessitating careful examination of study results. High rates of cocaine use and concomitant use of other substances have been reported across all socioeconomic classes (Griffith et al., 1994). However, children exposed prenatally to cocaine tend to be affected in different ways (Barone, 1994a), and the variations in effects depend on the frequency of cocaine use, route of administration, amount of the average dose, stage of fetal development, and the genetic susceptibility of the fetus (Lewis, 1991). Along these lines, research by Bateman, Ng, Hansen, and Heagarty (1993) has suggested that the media's portrayal of crack cocaine as more harmful than powder cocaine may have some basis in reality. They found that crack smoking results in a greater number and degree of problems (shortened gestation, lower fetal weight, smaller length and head circumference) than other forms of cocaine use. But because powder cocaine and crack cocaine are metabolized by the body in the same manner, the greater problems may be attributable to distinctive patterns of cocaine use rather than any chemical differences. Users of crack have a tendency to ingest greater quantities of cocaine, and perhaps have more irregular patterns of usage, compared with users of cocaine powder.

Although cocaine use in pregnancy has not been associated with any proven set of defects (Greider, 1995), the effects of prenatal exposure to alcohol and nicotine are well documented. Information about the detrimental impact of alcohol and tobacco may be more available to greater numbers of women due to the warning labels on cigarettes, beer, wine, and hard liquor. However, admonitions about the use of these substances during pregnancy are often undermined by the fact that alcohol and tobacco are both legal drugs, and many women falsely equate legality with safety.

A leading cause of mental retardation and birth defects in the United States is fetal alcohol syndrome (Scherling, 1994). Alcohol's effects include dysmorphogenesis (the development of ill-shaped or otherwise malformed body structures), growth abnormalities, and cognitive and language deficits. Several studies have found alcohol use and cigarette smoking during pregnancy to be associated with lower IQ scores and poorer language development and cognitive functioning (Fried & Watkinson, 1990; Streissguth, Barr, Sampson, Darby, & Martin, 1989). Cigarette smoking has also been associated with prenatal complications, low birth weight, and impairment in language and cognitive development (Fried & O'Connell, 1987; Gonzalez & Campbell, 1994). In fact, exposure to alcohol and cigarettes has been determined to have an equal or greater detrimental impact on the infant than exposure to cocaine (Richardson, Day, & McGauhey, 1993).

Little research has been conducted to examine the relative effects of different drugs used singly or simultaneously during pregnancy. However, some studies have found that fetal growth detriments are greater when cocaine is used in combination with other drugs—possibly due to heavier overall drug use, synergism with other substances, or the effects of the substances themselves (Bateman et al., 1993; Nulman et al., 1994; Singer, Arendt, Song, Warshawshy, & Kliegman, 1994). One major study that examined the effects of prenatal cocaine or cocaine and multiple drug use on the development of infants found that the drug-exposed children had significantly smaller head circumference at age 2 years than nondrug-exposed children (Chasnoff, Griffith, Freier, & Murray, 1992), but by age 3 years, there was no significant difference (Griffith et al., 1994). In addition, no individual drug exposure predicted small head size. By contrast, Joseph Jacobson et al. (1994) at Wayne State University were able to identify the unique effects of multiple substances on birth size in a prospective study. By using appropriate statistical controls, examinations of alcohol, smoking, opiates, and cocaine revealed that birth weight and length were related only to maternal alcohol use and smoking. Cocaine use was related only to gestational age, whereas head circumference was linked primarily to prenatal opiate and alcohol exposure (Jacobson et al., 1994).

Although many early studies attributed a variety of medical, behavioral, and learning problems to cocaine exposure, the children at risk are also susceptible to environmental factors that may affect physical, emotional, and social development (Barone, 1993). Over and above the effects of substance abuse, other variables, including nutrition, environment, and delivery date, can affect the overall health of a child. Within this context, women drug users have been found to differ from nondrug using women in a number of important ways. Substance abuse among women is considered a marker for many traits, including lifestyle, demographic characteristics, and socioeconomic status (Broekhuizen, Utrie, & Van Mullen, 1992; Richardson et al., 1993). Drug and alcohol addictions in women have also been linked with low self-esteem, domestic abuse, a history of sexual abuse, and a chaotic lifestyle (Broekhuizen et al., 1992). In addition, cocaine-using women tend to suffer from poor nutrition and overall health, a greater exposure to violence, and poor or unsanitary living conditions with greater risk of infections than other women (Greider, 1995; Scherling, 1994).

It is important that inadequate prenatal care has also been correlated with substance use, particularly with the use of cocaine, and may serve as an indication of substance abuse (Bibb et al., 1995; Fenton, McLaren, Wilson, Anderson, & Curry, 1993). Previous studies have suggested that women with few prenatal visits or those who initiate prenatal care late in the pregnancy tend to be younger, non-white, single women drug users of low socioeconomic status, who more often than not had nutritional deficits and inadequate health care (Funkhouser, Butz, Feng, McCaul, & Rosenstein, 1993; Richardson et al., 1993). Pregnant women from the nation's inner cities who were not involved in a prenatal care program have also been found to have significantly higher rates of hepatitis B and syphilis than patients actively participating in a medically supervised prenatal care program (Ernst, Romolo, & Nick, 1993; Silverman, Darby, Ronkin, & Wapner, 1991). Because of inadequate medical care, many pregnant addicts deliver prematurely, and characteristics of premature infants are not unlike characteristics of those exposed prenatally to crack cocaine (Barone, 1994a; Sexson, 1993).

Many times, studies of the effects of cocaine exposure have sampled pregnant women using multiple substances who have also had inadequate prenatal care. Within this context, it is uncertain whether unsatisfactory pregnancy outcomes resulted from the lack of medical care itself or whether other factors, such as drug abuse, were to blame (Richardson et al., 1993). With this in mind, a number of studies have documented the importance of appropriate prenatal care in improving both infant and maternal health (Randall, 1991; Richardson et al., 1993; Scholl, Hediger, & Belsky, 1994). In a study of indigent, pregnant drug abusers conducted at New York University Medical Center, it was demonstrated that so-called intensive prenatal care could be remarkably beneficial for pregnancy outcomes (Randall, 1991). The study included biweekly obstetric visits from enrollment to 36 weeks gestation, and 35 women participated. Routine prenatal laboratory procedures and urine testing to estimate maternal drug use were also performed. In addition, the women received counseling on nutrition, sexually transmitted diseases, and fetal development. The results of the study were dramatic. All of the pregnancies resulted in live births with no abnormalities observed, and only one infant was delivered prematurely; 4 women (11%) delivered low-birth-weight infants, which approximated the average rate of low-birth-weight infants in the entire hospital population (Randall, 1991). Support for the results of this study was provided by numerous other investigations of the benefits of prenatal care among drug-using women. Pregnancy outcomes of addicted women improved if they received prenatal care—both gestational age at delivery and birth weight were significantly better than in addicted women who received no prenatal care (Hawthorne & Maier, 1993). A further study found that women who used cocaine and also had adequate prenatal care did not experience a higher rate of obstetric complications when compared with a noncocaine-using control group (Richardson et al., 1993).

Similarly, the work of Broekhuizen and colleagues at the University of Wisconsin Medical School found that the adequacy of prenatal care affected pregnancy results more than drug use itself (Broekhuizen et al., 1992). Going further, in the largest study of its kind, 7,470 women who enrolled in prenatal care programs were monitored for drug use (Shiono et al., 1995). Of the 2.3% who used cocaine while pregnant, cocaine use was not correlated with preterm delivery, low birth weight, or small head circumference. Only cigarette smoking was found to increase the proportion of low-birth-weight infants. In fact, the authors estimated that 15% of the low-birth-weight infants could have been prevented if the mothers had not used cigarettes while pregnant (Shiono et al., 1995).

Although prenatal care has been shown to significantly improve pregnancy outcomes, the elements of prenatal care that are effective at reducing risk need to be assessed. Prenatal care may provide some of its benefit through prevention or early detection and treatment of maternal complications that occur during the period of gestation (Scholl et al., 1994). It is often an arduous task to separate the unique effects of cocaine exposure from those of other drugs or an otherwise unhealthy prenatal environment or maternal lifestyle (Scherling, 1994). What is certain, however, is that all of these factors affect children's health, social functioning, and well-being.

Richardson and Day (1994) have further suggested that the effects of cocaine on infant growth are an illusion. These researchers assert that the mother's lifestyle characteristics are more indicative of infant outcome than is her cocaine use. For example, in their study, the difference in birth weight between cocaine-exposed infants and nonexposed infants was found to be statistically significant (the difference did not occur by chance) at 307 grams. However, when the infants' gestational ages were taken into account, the weight difference between the infants of users and nonusers was reduced to a nonsignificant 128 grams. By also controlling for differences in tobacco and alcohol use between the two groups, the weight deviation was reduced to 82 grams. When the infants' races and genders were also taken into account, the weight discrepancy between the cocaine-exposed and nonexposed fell to only 33 grams. In sum,

Richardson and Day explained, "Preliminary data are presented to illustrate the thesis that it may not be cocaine per se that affects infant outcome (the illusion), but a multitude of factors including sociodemographic characteristics and the use of drugs (the reality)" (p. 29).

Indeed, the postnatal environment has been shown to be a crucial factor in development for all infants (Scherling, 1994). Perhaps two of the most important aspects of the postnatal environment that have been shown to affect child development are drug abuse and poverty in the household. Many mothers who abuse drugs during pregnancy continue to do so after birth and may enter treatment only when it is compulsory (Scherling, 1994). In addition, the treatment that is available may be inappropriate for the mother's particular psychological, social, and economic needs (Kumpfer, 1991). As such, many drug-exposed infants who return home to a drug-using environment after birth are at high risk for abuse and neglect (Rudigier, Crocker, & Cohen, 1990). In a recent study of drug-exposed 3-year-olds, 40% of the children whose parents continued to use drugs after birth had less than average language skills, whereas only 15% of the children whose parents were no longer using drugs reflected such limitations (Scherling, 1994). Another 1994 study found that drug-exposed children who continued to live in a drug-using household after birth experienced significant delays in verbal reasoning (Griffith et al., 1994). In addition, although all drug-exposed children (cocaine exposed and noncocaine exposed) in this study were rated by caregivers as displaying more destructive behaviors than non-drug-exposed children, cocaine alone was not found to predict aggressive behavior. The majority of the drug-exposed children in this study scored in the average range on intellectual abilities and displayed no significant behavior problems (Griffith et al., 1994).

Children Living in Poverty

Perhaps the most significant single predictor of developmental problems for children is the socioeconomic status of the family. In 1991, 21.8% of children in the United States were in families living below the poverty line (U.S. Bureau of the Census, 1992). African American and Latino children are more likely than other children to reside in low-income households, with 45.9% and 40.4%, respectively, living below the poverty line (U.S. Bureau of the Census, 1992). Poverty has a dramatic impact on parenting, home environment, family structure, child care, and access to resources (Huston, McLoyd, & Coll, 1994). Poor children are also at higher than average risk for health and nutrition problems, which may negatively affect their physical and cognitive development (Huston et al., 1994). The *Journal of the American Medical Association* reported that only 40% to 50% of 2-year-olds across the country are fully immunized and that the percentage is significantly lower among poor children (Bates, Fitzgerald, Dittus, & Wolinsky, 1994). Mothers living below the poverty line are less likely to begin immunizations for their children by 3 months of age and less likely to complete the immunization process (Bates et al., 1994), which places poor children at higher risk of contracting serious infections. Similarly, Newacheck and colleagues at the University of California-San Francisco Institute for Health Policy Studies reported significantly higher levels of middle-ear disease, skin lesions, and chronic illness among children from low-income families (Newacheck, Jameson, & Halfon, 1994).

Poor children are also particularly vulnerable to a significant health risk from lead exposure. Lead exposure has been found to be a potentially confounding factor in the low birth weights of cocaine-exposed newborns. An estimated 35% of poor, inner city, black children had elevated blood lead levels compared with only 5% of nonpoor, white children living outside of central cities (U.S. Department of Health and Human Services, 1994). It is not uncommon for cocaine users to be exposed to lead in the older, substandard housing associated with the conditions of poverty. Given this knowledge, Neuspiel, Markowitz, and Drucker (1994) hypothesized that cocaine-exposed fetuses would have experienced more lead exposure and that the lead or tobacco, or both, would partially explain any deficit in growth thought to be attributed to cocaine. These researchers found that growth detriments in cocaine-exposed newborns were indeed lessened after taking the influence of both lead and tobacco into consideration. Lead poisoning has traditionally been linked to high infant mortality, low birth weight, convulsions, failure to thrive, and delayed physical and mental development (Vimpani, 1995).

Lead exposure has also been implicated in infant seizures, irritability, lethargy, abdominal pain, and anemia (Lockitch et al., 1991; Vimpani, 1995). More subtle effects on neurological development, including auditory function, reaction time, word recognition skills, and behavioral disturbances, have also been observed (Vimpani, 1995). Recently, NIDA (1994) has also suggested that some health effects on newborns attributed in the past to cocaine use may have resulted from the presence of lead. Although lead is unlikely to be the sole source of developmental problems in children, the developing nervous system of an infant is extremely sensitive to lead toxicity, and previous research has demonstrated a neurotoxicological interaction between lead and cocaine that can affect cognitive development (Centers for Disease Control, 1991). In addition, IQ scores at age 5 years have been found to be significantly lower among children from low-income families at risk for lead exposure, compared with high-income, low-risk children (Duncan, Brooks-Gunn, & Klebanov, 1994; Vimpani, 1995).

Children from low-income families are also more likely to display significant behavioral problems than other children (Duncan et al., 1994; Newacheck et al., 1994). One 1994 study found that lower family economic status was associated with internalizing behaviors, such as fearfulness, sadness, anxiety, and depression, and with externalizing behaviors, such as temper tantrums and rage (Duncan et al., 1994). Similarly, other researchers reported 38% more behavioral problems on average among children from lower-income families than higher-income families (Newacheck et al., 1994). The most frequently reported problem behaviors reported in this study included antisocial behavior (cruel, mean, disobedient, not sorry for misbehaving, trouble getting along with others), hyperactivity, and social withdrawal. It is interesting that many of these same behaviors have frequently been observed in drug-exposed infants and have often been attributed to cocaine use. The findings of these studies reinforce the notion that the postnatal environment has a significant impact on infant development and should be examined in future studies of cocaine-affected infants.

Given the significant obstacles facing drug-exposed, poor infants, what are their prospects for the future? Early intervention appears to be a fundamental part of successful developmental outcomes for many drug-exposed or poor (or both) children. Intensive intervention programs in the first year after birth have been encouraging (Scherling, 1994). Drug-exposed infants enrolled in an educational program at Boston City Hospital all fell within the normal range on infant development tests at age 1 year (Zuckerman, 1991). Further research also established that crack-exposed children could be successfully integrated into active learning centers with nondrug-exposed children and reported that crack-exposed children adjusted well to a variety of classroom environments and did not require environments devoid of stimulation (Barone, 1993; Sautter, 1992).

In addition, a 1994 study reported that organized day care was positively associated with better reading and math skills among low-income children from low-quality home environments (Caughy, DiPietro, & Strobino, 1994). Participation in after-school child care programs has also been associated with improved academic skills and positive socioemotional development among low-income children (Posner & Vandell, 1994).

Postscript

Prenatal cocaine exposure has been debated at length but with little consensus or agreement. Are there really cocaine babies per se, or are these children affected by a complex set of factors? Going further, there are some who assert that the crack-baby crisis is in fact a myth advanced to fuel a sociopolitical agenda. Or as explained by one observer,

> The crack-baby myth was so powerful in part because it had something for everyone, whether one's ideological leanings called for enhancing public programs to meet the crisis, or for punishing the drug-addicted mothers seen as responsible for it. (Greider, 1995, p. 55)

Few methodologically sound, long-term studies examining the effects of prenatal cocaine exposure exist (Cole & Platzman, 1993; Gonzalez & Campbell, 1994). As such, researchers caution that although immediate deleterious effects of cocaine use on the infant may not be apparent, the possibility that consequences of exposure may surface later in life should not be discarded. Dr. Joseph Volpe (1992) of Harvard Medical School explains that adverse effects of cocaine exposure may have actually been downplayed because these effects may be too complex to ascertain. He has further suggested that the current tests and procedures used to examine the impact of cocaine on the fetus may not sufficiently evaluate the actual effects. In other words, the damaging effects of a mother's cocaine use on her child may have been underestimated simply because the advanced technology or knowledge required for complex diagnoses are unavailable.

There have, in fact, been numerous investigators who recognize that the effects of cocaine on the fetus are potentially significant. For example,

Given the knowledge of the devastating effects of crack-cocaine on adults, results from controlled animal studies, and retrospective postnatal studies of infants and children, it is generally accepted that acute and long-term effects of in-utero exposure to the drug (cocaine) on the human fetus are extremely serious, and in some cases will result in life-long multigenerational problems. (Scherling 1994, p. 9)

However, researchers agree that effects will vary from infant to infant depending on a variety of factors. More important, it is largely maintained that some, perhaps even many, of the children prenatally exposed to cocaine will experience few to no detrimental effects at all. And the longitudinal studies of prenatal cocaine exposure that are under way are in their early stages, and long-term developmental outcomes are not yet conclusive (Scherling, 1994). Thus, when examining the potential consequences of prenatal cocaine exposure and weighing the evidence, it is essential that one considers other factors that may have contributed to problematic outcomes. These factors include characteristics and lifestyle preferences of the mother—other illicit drug use, tobacco and alcohol use, socioeconomic status, nutritional intake, health condition, stress, and access to prenatal care.

In the final analysis, it has proven difficult to separate the prenatal effects of cocaine from other potentially negative influences on the fetus's and growing child's development. Nevertheless, the following chapter examines the most recent research on cocaine's effects on a woman's pregnancy and on her fetus and newborn and developing child.

Notes

1. More recently, NIDA estimates place the number of infants exposed to cocaine annually at 45,000 (Mathias, 1995).

2. Complete descriptions of placental abruption, microcephaly, and other possible adverse effects appear in Chapter 3.

3. Although cocaine seems to be abused equally in all socioeconomic strata (Bingol et al., 1987; Chasnoff & Griffith, 1989a), it is reported less frequently among pregnant women of higher socioeconomic status who can afford private obstetric care and who deliver in private hospitals and clinics, making it easier to conceal any evidence of substance abuse (Scherling, 1994).

3. The Effects of Prenatal Exposure to Cocaine

W hen cocaine is ingested—regardless of whether it is smoked, snorted, or injected—the effects of the drug include constriction of the blood vessels and irregular heartbeat. If the user is a pregnant woman, these actions reduce or interrupt the supply of nutrient-rich blood flowing to the fetus (Tronick & Beeghly, 1992; Woods, Plessinger, & Clark, 1987). Thus, not only does cocaine have the potential to complicate a woman's pregnancy but to affect her developing fetus as well. And because "maternal use equals fetal exposure" (Dixon, 1994, p. 136), recent research has focused on all phases of cocaine exposure as it relates to the fetus and infant. To date, much of the work has examined a broad range of developmental, behavioral, and cognitive problems that may emerge.

Complications During Pregnancy

Women who use cocaine may experience a variety of problems throughout the course of their pregnancies as well as during child-

birth. These complications have been reported to include spontaneous abortions, stillbirths, ruptured placentas, and premature labor
and delivery. Although cocaine use in pregnancy is considered a
major public health problem (Neuspiel & Hamel, 1991), it is not
fully clear whether the complications experienced by cocaine-using
mothers are direct or indirect effects of the drug, the result of other
maternal characteristics and behaviors, environmental factors, or a
combination of these.

Spontaneous Abortion and Stillbirth

Spontaneous abortions, more commonly referred to as *miscar-
riages,* usually occur early in pregnancy and result from abnormalities
of the fetus, factors in the maternal environment, or both. Oftentimes, spontaneous abortions occur even before a woman realizes
she is pregnant, and thus, it is difficult to determine incidence rates
of spontaneous abortion among the general public. It is even harder
to judge their frequency in cocaine users because women who use
drugs have less contact with health services (Robins & Mills, 1993).
Overall, however, general estimates suggest that more than 10% of
all pregnancies end in spontaneous abortion.

A study of 75 women who had used cocaine sometime during
pregnancy was conducted at the Perinatal Center for Chemical
Dependence in Chicago. It was determined that these cocaine-using
women were more likely than a group of nonusers to have spontaneous first-trimester abortions (Chasnoff, 1986/1987). Similarly, in
an examination of the health histories of cocaine-using and nonusing
pregnant women, it was found that those who were users of cocaine
had a significantly greater frequency of previous spontaneous abortions (Singer et al., 1994).

It is important to understand that estimates of spontaneous abortion due to drug use are likely to underestimate their actual occurrence, because they are often undetected unless medical assistance is
required. Moreover, even when they require medical attention, the
association with drug use is often missed (Robins & Mills, 1993).
Consequently, few studies exist that attempt to measure or explain
their occurrence in drug-using women.

Stillbirth refers to the birth of a fetus that died either before or
during delivery. Stillbirths can, for obvious reasons, be more directly
measured than spontaneous abortions. Burkett, Yasin, Palow, LaVoie,
and Martinez (1994) examined fetal outcomes at delivery for 905
multiethnic and multiracial inner-city pregnant cocaine-using women.

They found that, overall, 14% of the women gave birth to stillborn infants. The percentage of fetuses that were stillborn varied depending on whether the woman's pattern of cocaine bingeing was cyclical (5.0%), daily (16.4%), or erratic (20.5%). The erratic pattern of cocaine use was thought to have had the most traumatic impact on pregnancy. Women in this group had unpredictable crack bingeing habits, which often included exposure to higher concentrations of cocaine over long and sustained periods of time.

Placental Abruption

Placental abruption (known as *abruptio placentae* in medical terminology) is a severe complication of pregnancy where the placenta becomes detached from the wall of the uterus. Some of the complications associated with placental abruption are vaginal bleeding; fetal distress; rapid, painful labor; and blood clotting. Because this condition often results in severe hemorrhaging, it is a significant cause of maternal and fetal death. Placental abruption has been found to occur more often in women with high blood pressure, but in many cases, there is no explanation. This condition is not uncommon, occurring approximately once in every 200 births.

When a woman uses cocaine during the later stages of her pregnancy, evidence suggests that the drug may cause the uterus to contract and subsequently to initiate premature labor. If the contractions are intense, the placenta may separate from the uterus causing an abruption. Because the fetus is dependent on the oxygen delivered by the placenta, the infant will die unless rapid delivery via cesarean section occurs (Sexson, 1993). Research has suggested that cocaine use may indeed be associated with placental abruption. In a study of 361 cocaine-using mothers, it was determined that the rate of placental abruption was 7 times that of a control group of nondrug users (Bateman et al., 1993). Similarly, Dow-Edwards, Chasnoff, and Griffith (1992) found that 17% of the cocaine-using mothers in their study experienced placental abruption compared with only 1% of the cocaine-free mothers. And in a multicenter study of women attending prenatal clinics, cocaine use was found to be strongly associated with placental abruption. In fact, almost 11% of the women in this latter study who had used cocaine during pregnancy experienced placental abruption, as compared with 2.3% of those who did not (Shiono et al., 1995).

It is interesting, however, that other studies have found that the rate of placental abruption among cocaine users is not unlike that of nonusers. MacGregor et al. (1987), for example, found that the rates of placental abruption were not statistically different (7.1% for mothers who used cocaine and 1.4% for the control group). The researchers concluded, however, that the difference between the two groups was "clinically alarming" (p. 689).

Premature Birth

Medically, premature infants are those born before 37 weeks of gestation. Some predisposing factors associated with prematurity are multiple pregnancy, severe trauma to the mother or fetus, blood toxicity, and chronic disease, but in most cases, the cause is unknown. The incidence of prematurity is highest among women of low socioeconomic status, who are often suffering from inadequate nutrition and lack of prenatal care. Premature infants may have poor sucking reflexes, respiratory difficulties, and a variety of other problems.

Although many premature infants develop normally, complications from prematurity can result in death. According to National Center for Health Statistics (NCHS) data, in 1995, prematurity-low birth weight was one of the leading causes of death among infants in the United States. In 1991, it was the third leading cause of death for White infants and the major cause for Black infants (Singh & Yu, 1995). Maternal cocaine use has been found to be a possible factor in premature birth. The use of cocaine during the third trimester may induce a sudden onset of contractions within minutes to hours after ingestion of the drug. These contractions have the potential to induce preterm labor (Chasnoff, 1986/1987).

Several studies have shown that rates of preterm delivery are, in fact, quite high for women who use cocaine. For example, the risk of preterm delivery for cocaine-exposed infants at an inner-city hospital was found to be more than double that of nonexposed infants—32% of mothers with a history of cocaine use versus 14% of the nonusers (Bateman et al., 1993). Other research, furthermore, has yielded comparable findings (see Dow-Edwards et al., 1992; MacGregor et al., 1987). And last, it has been found that cocaine use, when compared with use of tobacco, alcohol, marijuana, and heroin, was the best predictor of prematurity (Singer et al., 1994).

When infants are born prematurely, they face a number of health problems. They are at greater risk of injury and illness than are full-term, normal-sized newborns (Lester & Tronick, 1994). The most common consequence of prematurity is respiratory distress syndrome (Sexson, 1993), a complication that requires the use of a ventilator to aid with breathing. If a ventilator is needed for a prolonged time, the infant may develop a chronic scarring of the lungs. Another potential consequence of premature birth is intraventricular hemorrhage, a condition that can damage the brain.

Despite these potential difficulties associated with cocaine exposure, most premature infants have a low risk of subsequent medical problems, and their development as they approach school age is comparable to that of full-term infants (Sexson, 1993). Along these lines, a study by Chasnoff and Griffith (1989) followed cocaine-exposed infants for 2 years and compared them with infants exposed to other drugs and with those who had had no illicit drug exposure. Each group was similar with regard to the mother's smoking history and social background, but the cocaine-exposed group was found to be the smallest at birth. However, by age 2 years, those exposed to cocaine had caught up, and the three groups were found to be equal in weight.

Effects on the Fetus

Cocaine enters the fetus rapidly after maternal use. As the drug passes through the placenta, it crosses the blood-brain barrier, potentially affecting the developing fetal brain and other organs and tissues (Mayes, 1992). Once in the fetus, cocaine has a longer half-life than it does in the mother. *Half-life* refers to the length of time required to reduce a drug level to one half of its initial value in the body. Cocaine has a longer half-life in the fetus than in the adult because the fetal liver is not fully developed and thus cannot eliminate the drug quickly and because the enzymes and fluids that are responsible for the breakdown of cocaine are decreased in women during pregnancy (Chasnoff, 1987; Ewing, 1992). The consequences of this exposure can include impaired fetal growth, low birth weight, and microcephaly (small head circumference), many of which are likely related to premature birth (Bateman et al., 1993).

Size at Birth

Newborns thought to be cocaine exposed have been described by the untrained observer as noticeably small in size compared with nonexposed infants. There is also a partial consensus in the medical and research communities as to the validity of these lay observations. Indeed, some researchers have found that approximately 25% of cocaine-exposed infants have experienced some form of growth retardation in utero (Fulroth, Phillips, & Durant, 1989). And furthermore, a lengthy report analyzing more than 100 clinical and research studies on the effects of prenatal exposure to drugs, submitted as a supplement to the *American Journal of Public Health,* concluded that,

> Nearly all of the available evidence indicates that cocaine-exposed babies are smaller than average at birth, in part because they are more often born premature. Studies have ruled out the possibility that the association between small babies and cocaine was the spurious (false) effect of smoking, lack of prenatal care, or an individual propensity to have babies of low birth weight. (Robins and Mills, 1993, pp. 8, 15)

There are many complications associated with low birth weight. Low-birth-weight infants are 40 times more likely to die in their first month than normal-weight infants; survivors are at an increased risk of lifelong disabilities, including mental retardation, cerebral palsy, and visual and hearing impairment (March of Dimes, 1992).

A newborn weighing less than 2500 grams or 5.5 pounds is typically considered to be low birth weight. Low birth weight of cocaine-exposed infants has been attributed to several causes. Studies have shown that a decrease in uterine blood flow from the ingestion of cocaine results in oxygen deficiency and decreased fetal nutrition. The consequence of these deficiencies is a fetus undergrown and small for gestational age, and hence, with a lower weight at birth (Sexson, 1993; Woods et al., 1987).

An alternative or supplemental explanation for low birth weight is proposed by Frank et al. (1990). These researchers associate cocaine use with reduced fat stores, suggesting that cocaine might alter nutrient transfer from the mother to the fetus or that cocaine might actually increase fetal metabolism or both. Similarly, cocaine may affect the mother's nutrition and metabolism thus interfering with the infant's growth. Cocaine, as with other stimulants, is known to cause a decreased appetite in its users. Crack-cocaine users in particular often use drugs for lengthy periods without eating (Inciardi et al., 1993). Specifically, research on cocaine-using mothers has shown that they weigh on average 7 kgs (about 15 pounds) less than nonusing mothers (Singer et al., 1994) and that 33% of pregnant daily users of cocaine weigh under 100 lbs (Burkett et al., 1994).

Other researchers have examined growth retardation and low birth weight as an outgrowth of the infants' gestational age. Gestational age refers generally to the amount of time a developing fetus spends in the mother's uterus after conception. Gestational age can be determined by uterine measurement, detection of fetal heart tones, and ultrasonographic information. For a normal pregnancy, the total period of gestation should be at least 37 weeks, which is the length of time from the first day of the mother's last menstrual period to the time of delivery. An infant born after 41 weeks of pregnancy is considered postmature.

Cocaine-exposed infants have been determined to have shorter gestational ages than nonexposed infants. Medical researchers have found that the average gestational age for newborns delivered by cocaine-using women was 37.1 weeks, whereas the average gestational age for those born to noncocaine-using women was 39.3 weeks (MacGregor et al., 1987). As mentioned earlier, cocaine is known to cause a decrease in uterine blood flow, which may result in the ftus being underdeveloped and small for gestational age (Sexson, 1993). Thus, a cocaine-exposed newborn can be delivered on time but may still be smaller than expected for an infant of the same gestational age.

Investigations of the actual birth weights of cocaine-exposed infants have indicated that these infants weigh less at birth than do nonexposed infants. In fact, the risk of low birth weight was found to be more than doubled in some studies. Although empirical data on this topic are scarce, one small study of cocaine-exposed infants detected a significant difference in the average birth weight between exposed infants (6.3 lbs.) and nonexposed infants (7.5 lbs; MacGregor et al., 1987). Going further, 23% of the cocaine-exposed infants were considered to be low birth weight (less than 5.5 lbs.), whereas only 4% of the nonexposed were similarly categorized. Data collected on infants delivered to a population of inner-city women in New York City likewise demonstrated that 31% of the cocaine-exposed infants were low birth weight, as compared with only 10% of those infants not exposed to cocaine or other illicit drugs (Bateman et al., 1993). Rates of admission to neonatal intensive care in this study were 15% for nonexposed infants and 24% for cocaine-exposed infants, with low birth weight cited as the primary reason for admission in both groups. Researchers attributed the infants' growth deficiencies to cocaine use by the mother, with larger growth deficits ascribed to heavier cocaine use.

Microcephaly

One of the few purported effects of maternal cocaine use on the fetus for which there is widespread agreement is microcephaly, or small head circumference (see Ewing, 1992). Microcephaly is associated with a smaller than normal brain size in the fetus, and infants with this condition often suffer from mental retardation. Chromosomal abnormalities, exposure to toxic stimuli (i.e., cocaine), chemical agents, maternal infection during prenatal development, or any trauma, especially during the third trimester of pregnancy, are thought to be potential causes of microcephaly.

One large-scale review of the literature on studies of pregnant women who use stimulants estimated that between 15% and 20% of all stimulant-exposed newborns are affected by microcephaly (Dixon, 1994). Small head circumference reported in cocaine-exposed infants may result from direct effects of the drug on decreased brain growth, from nutritional deficits, or both (Neuspiel & Hamel, 1991). One investigation attempted to accurately disentangle these effects by examining the mothers' nutritional conditions, use of other illicit drugs during pregnancy, smoking during pregnancy, and other variables (Handler, Kistin, Davis, & Ferre, 1991). Small head circumference was more common among the cocaine-exposed infants (16% vs. 6%) and was predicted by cocaine use alone. Although it is generally acknowledged that fetal growth retardation is associated with maternal nutritional deficits, fetal head growth in cases of maternal malnutrition is usually relatively normal. This knowledge provides some justification for the attribution of microcephaly specifically to prenatal cocaine use (Jacobson, Jacobson, & Sokol, 1994; Jacobson, Jacobson, Sokol, & Martier, 1994; Volpe, 1992).

Fetal Malformations

Alcohol has been found to be a teratogen and has been proven to cause congenital (defined as existing at birth, but not hereditary) abnormalities. A *teratogen* is an agent that causes severe fetal malformations, such as deformed or missing limbs or the distinct facial abnormalities seen in some children diagnosed with fetal alcohol syndrome. At present, the ability of any drug other than alcohol to cause congenital abnormalities is uncertain (Robins & Mills, 1993). Initially, cocaine was believed to be a teratogen as well, and some early studies of cocaine-exposed infants reported birth defects of the kidney, arms, and heart (Cherukuri et al., 1988). These adverse effects were thought to result from cocaine's action on maternal blood pressure, which serves to decrease blood flow to developing fetal tissues and organs (Zuckerman, 1993). Today, however, there is wider recognition that many early studies failed to ascertain any teratogenic properties specific to cocaine, when the effects of alcohol and other drug use were removed (Ewing, 1992). The stability in the number of malformed infants born in the United States every year, despite the crack epidemic of the past decade, provides some anecdotal evidence against the argument that cocaine is a teratogen (Robins & Mills, 1993).

The Cocaine-Exposed Infant

Given the large body of literature on the effects of prenatal cocaine exposure, one might assume that there is a typical profile or symptomatology among such infants. However, the expectation of a deformed infant with a distinct facial appearance experiencing frequent seizures and other overt symptoms associated with drug withdrawal does not appear to be so (Sexson, 1993). In fact, the majority of cocaine-exposed infants are delivered without complication and born without apparent medical problems (Richardson & Day, 1994). However, when an infant born to a cocaine-using mother does experience medical difficulties, it has typically been born prematurely, often with a history of a ruptured placenta, and is small for gestational age (Sexson, 1993). These newborns may display abnormal crying patterns, may have sleep dysfunctions, and may respond erratically to stimuli (DiPietro, Seuss, Wheeler, Smouse, & Newlin, 1995; Lester et al., 1991). They may also have poor psychomotor ability that includes abnormal reflexes and imbalanced muscle tone (Dow-Edwards et al., 1992).

Sudden Infant Death Syndrome

Sudden infant death syndrome (SIDS), sometimes referred to as *crib death,* is the unexpected death of an apparently healthy infant within 6 months to 1 year of birth. SIDS deaths occur for unexplained reasons while the infant is sleeping. Proposed causes of SIDS are poor diet, respiratory defects, or viral infection, among many other possibilities. SIDS occurs more often in boys than in girls, in the winter months, in infants who have recently had minor illnesses, and with mothers who receive little prenatal care, who smoke and are drug dependent, or both.

Worldwide, SIDS is the most common cause of death in children between 2 weeks and 1 year of age; however, in the United States, the overall incidence of SIDS is relatively rare. For example, the rate of SIDS deaths in the U.S. population, according to 1995 data from the National Center for Health Statistics, was 86.9 per 100,000 live births. However, in some studies, rates of SIDS among cocaine-exposed infants have been found to be somewhat higher.

Early research suggested that a link existed between cocaine exposure and susceptibility to SIDS. In a small study of 66 infants exposed to cocaine prenatally, 10 were subsequently diagnosed as dying from SIDS—a rate more than triple that of samples of heroin-exposed and methadone-exposed infants (Chasnoff, 1986). A more recent study followed 224 infants, 105 of which were cocaine exposed and 119 of which were nonexposed infants. After 12 months, there had been four SIDS deaths, and all had occurred to infants who were cocaine exposed. It was concluded that cocaine use is a so-called marker for increased risk of SIDS (Porat, Brodsky, Giannetta, & Hurt, 1994), although the authors did indicate that the deaths could have resulted from other organic or environmental causes. Many of the mothers had received inadequate or no prenatal care and had also used alcohol and tobacco throughout their pregnancies, thus making cause and effect relationships difficult to establish. By contrast, other studies have found no increased risk of SIDS among cocaine-exposed infants (Bauchner et al., 1988; Fulroth, Durand, Nicjerson, & Espinoza, 1989).

Determining the risk of SIDS among infants who have been prenatally exposed to cocaine is difficult because many of the sociodemographic characteristics and health behaviors of the mother are also independently associated with SIDS (Bauchner et al., 1988). For example, other risk factors associated with SIDS are poverty, use of tobacco or opiates, and being African American. Many of the women in studies of cocaine use during pregnancy share just those characteristics and behaviors.

Along these lines, there may be other causes of SIDS that are not necessarily related to fetal drug exposure. There is the possibility that an infant may develop some of the risk factors associated with SIDS if exposed to cocaine after birth. The following excerpt is part of the case study of a 1-month-old infant who was likely exposed to crack smoke:

A 36-day-old female was brought to the emergency room after having had several episodes of apnea on that day. Stimulation was required to revive the baby during each episode. During some of the episodes the infant experienced vomiting, eye rolling, and limpness. Her urine drug screening was positive for significant levels of cocaine metabolites as was the mother's. (Okoruwa, Shah, & Gerdes, 1995, p. 449)

Overall, studies find no particular agreement as to whether there is an increased incidence of SIDS among cocaine-exposed infants. Moreover, a comprehensive review of the SIDS literature offers a similar conclusion (Barton, Harrigan, & Tse, 1995).

Neurological Problems

Cocaine is a powerful central nervous system stimulant with lasting neurobehavioral effects. Because cocaine can directly alter brain formation, fetal blood flow, and maternal nutrition, cocaine use may contribute to a biologically based vulnerability to neurodevelopmental impairments (Mayes, 1992). Thus, the development of a cocaine-exposed fetus into a healthy infant and child may be compromised. Potential manifestations of cocaine exposure, such as excessive crying or heightened reactivity to light and touch, have been observed in some infants thought to be drug exposed. More subtle neurobehavioral problems in the infant and growing child, such as slight delays in language development or intelligence, are difficult to measure even by medical and research experts.

Indeed, it has been difficult to demonstrate long-term behavioral, cognitive, and language problems in children who were exposed prenatally to cocaine (Mentis & Lundgren, 1995). Because prenatal cocaine exposure was not widely recognized or researched until the mid-1980s, the study of neurological dysfunction in cocaine-exposed infants and children has but a short history. Consequently, the continued study of neonatal functioning is necessary to confirm or refute general clinical impressions of cocaine-exposed infants.

Assessing Neurological Complications in Infants

The most persistent clinical impressions of cocaine-exposed infants involve sleep dysfunctions, irregularities in response to stimuli, and excessive crying and fussiness (DiPietro et al., 1995). These symptoms are believed by both the media and general public to be

the main effects of cocaine-exposure in young infants and are assumed to be related to cocaine withdrawal. However, rather than
suffering from withdrawal, the infant may still be experiencing the
direct effects of the mother's recent cocaine use (Neuspiel & Hamel,
1991; Schneider et al., 1989). Interestingly, some studies suggest
that cocaine-exposed infants are more easily aroused or provoked
than nonexposed infants, whereas other studies have found that
cocaine-exposed infants are actually more difficult to stimulate. It
has been proposed that infants in the former group are experiencing
the effects of recent maternal cocaine ingestion, while infants in the
latter group are exhibiting behavior indicative of the chronic effects
of maternal cocaine use on infants' growth (Lester, et al., 1991).

There are several tools that researchers and clinicians use to
evaluate the neurological effects of prenatal cocaine exposure. One
of these is the Brazelton Neonatal Behavioral Assessment Scale
(NBAS), a neurobehavioral scale used to measure the interactive
abilities and neurological status of both "normal" (nonexposed)
infants and drug-exposed infants up to 28 days of life. Another
assessment tool is the Bayley Scales of Infant Development (BSID),
employed in the evaluation of the mental, behavioral, and psychomotor development of infants ranging in age from 2 months to 2.5
years. The BSID measures perception, memory, and vocalization on
the mental scale; sitting, stair climbing, and manual manipulation
on the motor scale: and attention span, social behavior, and persis-
tence on the behavioral scale. Additional tests have been derived for
the specific purpose of assessing neurological problems in cocaine-
exposed infants, and others have been borrowed from their primary
function of evaluating infants exposed to other drugs, such as heroin.

Studies of cocaine-exposed infants tested with the NBAS have
yielded varying results. Newborns in one study suffered from decreased interactive skills, had short attention spans, and resorted to
either frantic crying or sleeping to shut themselves off from overstimulation (Dow-Edwards et al., 1992). Other adverse neurobehavioral manifestations of cocaine that have been reported include brief
tremors usually lasting less than 24 hours (Bateman et al., 1993).

As with the NBAS, evaluations done of cocaine-exposed infants
with the BSID have reported contradictory results. Chasnoff and
Griffith (1989b) tested infants who were exposed to cocaine and
compared these infants with those exposed to alcohol or marijuana
only and to infants with no drug exposure. Results indicated that
the cocaine-exposed infants showed no developmental delays on the
BSID.

Additional assessments of cocaine-exposed infants' visual-information processing and developmental progress demonstrated increased arousal in response to stimuli, which may exceed optimal levels for sustaining attentional and information processing capacities (Mayes, Bornstein, Chawarska, & Granger, 1995). In other words, infants that are prone to irritability and distress may have more difficulty learning skills and mastering tasks. With regard to the BSID evaluations, cocaine-exposed infants showed a comparatively depressed performance in psychomotor (muscular activity) development but fell into normal levels in terms of mental development.

Overall, it appears that evidence of adverse effects of prenatal cocaine exposure using the NBAS and BSID is inconclusive. Mentis and Lundgren (1995) have suggested that explicit conclusions are difficult to reach and that research results must be interpreted cautiously because the measures used to evaluate developmental outcomes may not be sufficiently sensitive to identify all possible problems. In addition, certain problems may only manifest at later stages of development, so tests such as the NBAS and BSID may be inadequate.

The Neonatal Abstinence Scale (NAS) was developed to describe characteristics of withdrawal syndromes among opioid-exposed infants but is sometimes used to assess cocaine-exposed infants. At least one study has found higher NAS scores (indicating more withdrawal symptoms) for infants exposed to both cocaine and an opiate than for those exposed to either cocaine or an opiate alone (Fulroth, Durand, et al., 1989), whereas another found no indication of withdrawal based on the NAS with cocaine-exposed infants (Doberczak et al., 1991). As is the case with other instruments used to measure the effects of cocaine exposure, the NAS scale may not be sensitive enough to assess cocaine's effects (Zuckerman, 1993).

In studying the neurological problems of cocaine-exposed newborns and infants, it has proven difficult to gauge the differences between infants born with very low birth weight due to a mother's use of cocaine and infants who are born with low birth weight for other reasons. That is, what proportion of the problems experienced by cocaine-exposed infants are directly related to low birth weight per se? One study that examined this issue looked at infants weighing less than 2500 grams that were similar with respect to gestational age, gender, and ethnicity. Results indicated that the cocaine-exposed group exhibited consistently poorer performances on tests at age 4 weeks than did nonexposed prematures, specifically in the areas of interaction, motor maturity, self-quieting, and ability to respond to stimuli. Thus, there is some evidence that the effects of cocaine are independent of birth weight (VandenBerg et al., 1994).

Cognitive Development

As cocaine-exposed infants grow older, another potential indicator of neurological impairment is delayed cognitive development. *Cognitive development* refers to the manner in which knowledge is acquired and information is processed. Some of the areas included in tests of an infant's cognitive development are language skills, literacy, memory, and intelligence levels.

In fact, problems in these areas were detected in a study of 35 infants exposed in utero to a variety of drugs, including cocaine. These infants were compared with 35 infants who were not drug exposed, and long-term follow-ups were conducted at 2.5 and 5.5 years of age. The drug-exposed children tended to score lower than the nonexposed group on all general intelligence and language tests, leading the authors to conclude that at preschool age, the drug-exposed children were functioning at a lower cognitive level than the control group (van Baar & de Graaff, 1994).

This conclusion seemed to be validated by similar studies that found significantly lower scores on tests measuring verbal comprehension and expressive language among cocaine-exposed children (Mentis & Lundgren, 1995; Nulman et al., 1994). There was no difference, however, in IQ levels between the cocaine-exposed children and a comparison group. Because the mothers of these children were matched on important criteria, such as IQ and socioeconomic status (two factors thought to strongly predict the home environment of the child), the question of whether prenatal cocaine exposure itself leads to negative outcomes was addressed. Within this context, the authors concluded that "this is the first study to document that intrauterine exposure to cocaine is associated with measurable and clinically significant toxic neurological effects, independent of postnatal home environmental confounders" (Nulman et al., 1994, p. 1591).

However, as is the case for research in many controversial areas, comparable examinations of the neurodevelopmental effects of cocaine exposure have produced results that contradict those of the aforementioned studies. Cognitive assessments using general cognitive, verbal performance, quantitative, and memory scales found no statistically significant differences between children who had been cocaine exposed and those that had not (Hawley, Halle, Drasin, & Thomas, 1995).

Going further, Diane Barone (1994b) examined the reading and writing skills of 26 cocaine-exposed children ranging in age from 1 to 7 years old. All of the children were being raised in stable foster homes, which was important to ensure that literacy behavior was not hampered by dysfunctional family environments. Although there were some noticeable delays, most children who were prenatally exposed to cocaine "were developing in literacy patterns that were similar to children who had not been prenatally exposed" (p. 311).

Other studies have found that outcomes for substance-exposed children in terms of cognitive development may vary according to factors in the home environment. For example, prenatal cocaine exposure was found to have a significant negative impact on verbal reasoning in 3-year-olds (independent of other drugs of exposure), but children most likely to display these verbal problems were those being raised in a home where drugs continued to be used (Griffith et al., 1994). This finding was reinforced by a similar piece of research that reported no differences in language delays between the drug-exposed and nonexposed children, leading the authors to conclude that these problems could not be attributed specifically to prenatal cocaine exposure. Instead, they may be due to negative effects of the caretaking environment (Malakoff, Mayes, & Schottenfeld, 1994). Thus, it appears that adverse effects of cocaine can be ameliorated by a stable environment but may be exacerbated by an unstable one.

In sum, there are data suggesting that prenatal cocaine exposure does affect neurological functioning and is manifested by inappropriate response to stimuli, attentional impairments, language difficulties, and other learning problems. However, the results were inconsistent, with some data suggesting that problems, if they were evident, were slight and could be counteracted in the proper home environment. And although research has demonstrated neurobehavioral differences between cocaine-exposed and nonexposed infants, it appears that as the children get older the, differences lessen. In fact, there is some evidence that suggests that a number of the reported dysfunctions of cocaine-exposed infants are no longer apparent by age 6 months (Mayes, 1992). Long-term evaluations of developmental outcomes in infants may help to clarify some of the issues surrounding the effects of prenatal cocaine exposure.

There is the hope and possibility that early neurodevelopmental dysfunctions in cocaine-exposed infants can be partially or completely ameliorated. The newborn brain may be able to adapt and compensate for at least some of the biological changes it has withstood (Zuckerman, 1993). Indeed, the infant and young child's brain has a unique plasticity, giving it the ability to recover from or overcome prenatal insult. Together, both brain plasticity and adequate caretaking may be able to compensate for some or all of the consequences of prenatal cocaine exposure (Mayes, 1992).

Social and Environmental Influences on Development

Most researchers agree that the postnatal home environment is crucial in that it can serve to either mitigate or potentiate and magnify the effects of prenatal cocaine exposure (Scherling, 1994). However, a long-standing bias in the research community (influenced in part by funding and public policy issues) has been that the cognitive and intellectual effects of cocaine exposure are of primary importance (Lester & Tronick, 1994). But recently, the study and importance of noncognitive outcomes, such as socioemotional development, parent-child relationships, and peer interaction, have come to the forefront. The overriding element in these interpersonal outcomes is the influence of the environment.

Often, the residences of those women for whom prenatal drug-use data are available are not optimal places for rearing children. Typically, they are single-parent homes located in lower socioeconomic neighborhoods where poverty flourishes (Sexson, 1993). In addition, the mother may continue to use drugs after giving birth and may spend less time caring for her infant. This could easily affect her parenting skills and, in some cases, may lead to abuse and neglect. In addition, the infants who are experiencing adverse effects of cocaine use may be more difficult to manage, potentially aggravating the overall situation (Mayes, 1992).

Whether reports of problematic socioemotional behaviors are a result of stress and anxiety levels among cocaine-using mothers or whether cocaine exposure specifically affects an infant's temperament and behavior is unclear (Edmondson & Smith, 1994; Singer et al., 1995). Either scenario is troubling, however, given that mothers need to establish a warm, empathic relationship with their infants and that psychological distress may impair a mother's ability to respond consistently to a child's needs. The coupling of this problem with decreased responsiveness, communicativeness, or both on the part of the infant produces less than optimal early caregiver-infant interaction and indirectly affects developmental outcome (Edmondson & Smith, 1994).

Continued Maternal Drug Use

Barry Zuckerman (1993) has offered the following explanation of drug addiction's impact on parenting:

> Central to the idea of addiction is the loss of control over the use of a substance and compulsive preoccupation despite the consequences. All aspects of the self are affected—the physical, the psychological, and the spiritual. With addicted women, their primary relationship is with their drug of choice, not with their children. Dysfunctional interactions (between the mother and infant) may interfere with an infant's ability to recover from a biological vulnerability caused by prenatal drug exposure. (p. 40)

Empirical evidence of this phenomenon was detected by researchers who found that crack cocaine acted to decrease mothers' attentiveness and their efforts to be appropriate role models for their children (Kearney, Murphy, & Rosenbaum, 1994). During in-depth interviews with crack-using mothers, one woman explained that crack made "the (mothering) responsibilities kind of fade out little by little" and stated further that, "the drug had me not caring" (Kearney et al., 1994, p. 354). It was common for many of these women to go on intense crack binges lasting hours or days, exhausting all of their financial resources and allowing for limited or no care of their children. Furthermore, even those women undergoing treatment for addiction have been shown to provide less adequate or stable home environments; their children moved frequently, had significantly less contact with their fathers, and had been placed in foster homes at much higher rates than were children of nonaddicted mothers (Hawley et al., 1995).

Abuse and Neglect

Prenatal exposure to cocaine has been found to be associated with maltreatment during infancy and early childhood. At a Chicago area hospital, records were reviewed for all infants born in a 5-year period who were exposed prenatally to illicit drugs, with the predominate drug of exposure being cocaine (Jaudes, Ekwo, & Van Voorhis, 1995). These records were compared with the State Child Registry, which contains information on all reports and investigations of allegations of child abuse and neglect. Of the 513 newborns who were prenatally exposed to drugs, 155 were reported as victims of abuse and 102 of these reports were substantiated. Neglect was the most common form of maltreatment, affecting 74% of the 102 children, and physical injury was recorded for 16% of the children. When rates of maltreatment from this study were compared with overall child abuse rates in the same area of Chicago during the same period, it was determined that children who were prenatally exposed to drugs were 2 to 3 times more likely to be victims of abuse and neglect than were nonexposed children.

Other studies have substantiated the claim that drug-exposed infants may be at an increased risk for maltreatment. At an urban Connecticut hospital, for example, researchers studied two groups of infants (47 cocaine-exposed and 47 nonexposed) to determine the occurrence of maltreatment, defined as physical or sexual abuse or neglect, during the first 2 years of life (Wasserman & Leventhal, 1993). By age 24 months, 23% of the children identified as cocaine exposed had been maltreated compared with only 4% of the comparison group.

Alternatively, maternal substance abuse has not been shown to predict neglectful parenting in other groups of women. Developmental assessments, interviews with the mothers, and observations of mother-child interactions during home visits failed to demonstrate any link between the developmental status of children and maternal substance use or caregiving adequacy. Adequacy of caregiving was also not related to the children's cognitive, motor, or expressive language development in this study (Harrington, Dubowitz, Black, & Binder, 1995).

Postnatal Exposure to Cocaine

As noted earlier, cocaine use during pregnancy typically continues after the birth of the child. If the mother is using cocaine in the home, there is a possibility that her infant or child will be exposed to it. As such, it is not uncommon for the children of crack-using parents to be exposed to toxic secondhand smoke. In a urinalysis of 250 children under age 5 years who entered an inner-city emergency room for the treatment of various ailments, for example, cocaine metabolites were found in 2.4% of the specimens (Kharasch, Glotzer, Vinci, Weitzman, & Sargent, 1991). And at the emergency department of the Children's Hospital of Michigan, cocaine was present in the urine of more than 5% of the 460 children aged 5 and below who underwent routine urinalysis as part of their treatment for such pediatric complaints as crying, fever, and diarrhea (Rosenberg, Meert, Knazik, Yee, & Kauffman, 1991).

Passive crack smoke inhalation was also thought to have caused or contributed to seizures and other neurological symptoms in four hospitalized children in New York City (Bateman & Heagarty, 1989). The following is a section of the patient report of an infant exposed to the secondhand crack smoke of her adult caretaker:

> A 3½-month-old girl was brought to our emergency ward because of the sudden onset of abnormal movements. These consisted of 30 second episodes of repetitive protruding of the tongue, choking, arching of the back, and brief jerking of both hands accompanied by a blank stare. Cocaine was isolated from the infant's urine. (Bateman & Heagarty, 1989, p. 25)

The infant was subsequently hospitalized for evaluation of the seizure, and 6 months after admission (and removal from her drug-using caretaker and placement with her grandmother), she had no further seizure activity. Neurological examination results, growth, and developmental progress were also normal.

Breast-feeding has been found to be a potential source of continued cocaine exposure from mother to infant through maternal milk. Because mothers who breast-feed commonly feed their infants 6 to 12 times in a 1-day period, cocaine exposure in this form can be frequent and substantial. In fact, researchers who have analyzed breast milk for drugs have found that cocaine concentrations in breast milk could reach extremely high levels. The concentration of cocaine in breast milk could be 20 times that of the mother's blood, leading to toxic infant blood concentrations (Dickson et al., 1994). The following case report of a 2-week-old infant whose mother used cocaine intranasally just prior to breast-feeding illustrates the possible effects of this type of cocaine exposure:

> The infant was brought to the emergency room with signs of cocaine intoxication: vomiting, diarrhea, hypertension, unfocused and dilated pupils, extreme irritability, and tremors. When tested, cocaine and its metabolites were found to persist in the mother's breast milk for approximately 48 hours after her last cocaine use. (Chasnoff, 1987; Chasnoff, Lewis, & Squires, 1987)

When cocaine is used in the home, there is the additional danger that it will be accessible to a child living at the residence. For

example, the *New York Times* recently reported a case in which an
11-month-old girl died of a heart attack after having been fed crack
by her 2-year-old brother ("Baby Fed Crack," 1995). The brother
apparently found the drug in his house, because it was part of his
mother's supply. The mother was charged with child abuse resulting
in death and possession and dealing of crack. These and other legal
issues surrounding the use of drugs by pregnant women and women
with children is examined in more detail in Chapter 4.

The Cocaine-Exposed Child in School

How children who were prenatally exposed to cocaine perform in
school is an area of current interest and of great controversy. There
has been much speculation about the difficulties that cocaine-
exposed children would face as they approached school age and,
subsequently, whether they should be taught in separate classrooms
designed to meet their special needs. The media, in particular, raised
fear levels in many communities with regard to cocaine-exposed
children entering school. Newspaper headlines announced, "Crack
Babies in School: They Will Deplete Resources and Test Compas-
sion" (Rist, 1990) and "As Drug Babies Grow Older, Schools Strive
to Meet Their Needs" (Trost, 1989). It is possible that the negative
assumptions made about cocaine-exposed children and their intellectual abilities have been especially damaging because some educators and parents believe this to be a certainty.

Within this context, it may be helpful to examine some common
beliefs regarding the schooling of cocaine-exposed children. To
follow are two myths that have been accepted by much of the lay
public and childhood educators as well:

> Myth 1—All children who are prenatally exposed to crack or other forms
> of cocaine are affected in similar ways and require intensive school
> intervention.
>
> Myth 2—Children who have been prenatally exposed to crack or other
> forms of cocaine require classrooms that have limited physical and
> social stimulation. (Barone, 1994, p. 67)

Given the overarching nature of such statements, it is important
that these claims be examined systematically. One such study attempted to measure the behaviors of children who were prenatally
exposed to cocaine and those who were not within the context of a
specialized preschool designed for children at risk. The results of

observations and assessments indicated that there were no statistically significant differences between the groups on many of the behavioral variables. The many behavioral and developmental similarities between the two groups of children studied raises the possibility that prenatal cocaine exposure may be less deleterious to development than we have been led to expect (Rotholz, Snyder, & Peters, 1995). Similarly, other researchers have reported like outcomes:

> Educators and clinicians may well feel heartened that the language and cognitive development of the crack-exposed children in this investigation did not differ from that of their Head Start (nonexposed) peers. In fact, the finding of so few group differences contradicts the widespread perception that prenatal cocaine exposure causes significant developmental disabilities. (Hawley et al., 1995, p. 375)

Some anecdotal accounts of educators who work with the cocaine exposed do report definite obstacles to learning for the cocaine exposed. The most common symptoms of drug-exposed children described in these accounts include attention deficit disorder, poor coordination, hyperactivity, low tolerance levels, unpredictability, and poor memory. An early-education teacher depicts her experience with a cocaine-exposed 5-year-old student in her kindergarten classroom:

> At first glance, Carl seemed small for his age, a bit thin, and noticeably hyperactive. In time he would prove to be a little powder keg of problems: inattentive, lacking in motor coordination, frustrated, and aggressively demanding of my attention. He tried hard to meet the challenges that school presented to him, but he always seemed acutely aware that he was not on the same wavelength as the rest of us. (Gregorchik, 1992, pp. 709-710)

Some teachers, because they have been told to expect failure in cocaine-exposed children, may see problems when they do not really exist. The adoptive mother of Daniel, a young boy who was exposed to crack prenatally, illustrates this point:

> The school knew [about his drug exposure] and it was written up in all the evaluations. Everything was related to his history. At two, he could count up to 20. He was learning how to count in Spanish by age three. He knew his alphabet. But, the school reports were absolutely horrifying. I mean, it wasn't the same child. According to them, he couldn't repeat two numbers consecutively, he couldn't turn the pages of a book, he

couldn't hold a pair of scissors. I mean, there was nothing this child could do. And that's because they *knew*. (Greider, 1995, p. 56)

Last, it is important to remember that learning, developmental, and behavioral problems may not be directly related to a mother's use of cocaine during pregnancy but may instead be due to a number of other factors. A positive approach to the education of cocaine-exposed children is regarded by many to be the only answer. As researcher Diane Barone (1995) explains, "Educators must move beyond using a single variable to explain a child's behavior; teachers must realize the fact that the child was prenatally exposed to drugs is not in itself an explanation for the child's learning" (p. 52).

Postscript

One factor that significantly complicates research on cocaine exposure but is inherent in each of the studies discussed is the method by which a woman or her newborn (or both) is screened for drug use. The typical screening processes either chemically test for the presence of cocaine metabolites in the urine or rely on the mother's self-report about her drug use. From urinalysis results or self-reported interview data, it is determined whether an infant is indeed cocaine exposed. The newborn is generally tested at birth or shortly after birth using urine or meconium (excrement in the fetal intestinal tract discharged at birth) screens. In the vast majority of cases, however, cocaine exposure goes undetected because these tests are not routinely performed in most hospitals.

Consequently, the potential for inaccurate determinations of cocaine use is considerable. Current urine tests are capable of accurately detecting cocaine metabolites in the mother within 2 to 3 days of usage. Similarly, urine screening of infants at birth is only accurate within 3 to 5 days of exposure. Furthermore, pregnant women may fail to report their drug use, perhaps even more so than nonpregnant women. One 1995 study illustrates the case in point—more than 90% of women who tested positive for cocaine had denied using the drug (see Shiono et al., 1995). Taking all of this into account, it is quite possible that cocaine-exposed infants born to mothers who denied drug use or who abstained from use several days prior to delivery (or testing) may in fact have been exposed to cocaine. This occurrence may serve to mask cocaine's actual effects (Bateman et al., 1993).

As alluded to earlier, there is a further issue to consider regarding screening for drug use. First, it is not a standard procedure in most medical establishments to test all mothers for drug use or all newborns for drug exposure. A few inner-city clinics conduct routine drug testing, but this is the exception rather than the rule. It appears that many clinics and hospitals do not have specific guidelines regarding who should get tested and under what circumstances. Many medical facilities have informal procedures that initiate testing only for infants who are born prematurely or who cry excessively. Similarly, testing of mothers may only be seen as necessary in cases where the mother "acts strangely," has had no prenatal care, or evidences a sexually transmitted disease.

Along these lines, there appears to be a correlation between a newborn's size at delivery and subsequent screening for drug use. This is plausible because doctors may be more likely to ask mothers of low-birth-weight infants about their drug use in an effort to explain the retarded growth (Robins & Mills, 1993). In addition, anecdotal reports indicate that when asked about how they can distinguish cocaine-exposed prematures from so-called normal prematures, nurses, obstetricians, and pediatricians frequently explain that cocaine-exposed newborns appear very small for what should be their normal gestational age. Otherwise, the absence of a distinct physical appearance in cocaine-exposed infants makes routine detection by physical examination virtually impossible (Sexson, 1993).

4. Prenatal Cocaine Use and the Prosecution of Pregnant Addicts

Prenatal maternal conduct and the subsequent rights of the fetus have endured as legal issues for more than 100 years. Civil actions involving fetal rights emerged as early as 1884 when a pregnant woman fell on a defective highway, resulting in the premature birth and eventual death of her fetus (*Dietrich v. Inhabitants of Northampton,* 1884). She was convicted of wrongful death and negligence, although the decision was ultimately overturned by the United States Supreme Court on the basis that the fetus could not be considered a legal person. Substance abuse among pregnant women, however, did not surface in the legal arena until considerably later; indeed, the first known attempt at the criminal prosecution of a pregnant drug user occurred in the late 1970s, and the application of civil sanctions involving parental neglect statutes began in 1980. But it was the emergence of cocaine, and specifically crack cocaine in the mid-1980s, that spawned the state's interest in the prosecution of pregnant drug users. As noted in earlier chapters, during this period, there was a growing body of research and numerous sensationalized media reports documenting the perils of cocaine exposure for the fetus. The public's increasing awareness of the issue, the conservative political climate, and drug control strategies that emphasized personal responsibility resulted in the development of public policies aimed at punishing, rather than treating, women who violated so-called fetal rights and exposed their unborn infants to cocaine.

By the closing years of the 1980s, women accused of illicit drug use during pregnancy, and those who gave birth to drug-exposed infants, were subject to a variety of criminal and civil actions—for neglect, delivery of drugs to a minor, child abuse and endangerment, and sometimes manslaughter and attempted murder (Sherman, 1988; Terry, 1996). Within such a context, much of this closing chapter examines the range of these criminal prosecutions and civil actions, followed by discussions of the constitutionality of punitive state intervention and the consequences of these actions on public policy and maternal drug use.

The Courts and Pregnant Drug Users

The campaign to combat prenatal drug use in the United States has focused on punitive rather than rehabilitative intervention, and the public policy battle has occurred under the auspices of the criminal justice system rather than through social welfare programs. Jurisdictions have initiated both criminal and civil actions, and in many cases, a combination of the two. In general, criminal prosecutions are a phenomenon of the post-Reagan era of the late 1980s and early 1990s. Almost without exception, criminal prosecutions of women who engaged in prenatal substance use have not stood up in the face of legal challenges (Center for Reproductive Law and Policy [CRLP], 1993; Paltrow, 1992). Unfortunately, however, many of the women charged under various criminal and civil statutes have lacked the resources to pursue court challenges and have received sentences as an outgrowth of court actions that were (and are), for all intents and purposes, unconstitutional and largely inapplicable in the face of state legislative guidelines.

During the last few years, some of these cases have proceeded to state appellate courts, although none has yet reached the United States Supreme Court. Although most actions taken by the state have not survived legal challenge, the courts have been hesitant to dismantle the state's apparent interest in protecting the fetus and holding the mother accountable for prenatal conduct that potentially causes harm. Instead, most appellate courts have overturned convictions on the basis that state action violated the initial intent of the legislature.

Criminal Prosecutions

One of the most striking aspects of the public concern over the issue of prenatal substance abuse was the speed with which states sought to make prenatal drug ingestion a criminal, as opposed to a public health or social welfare, issue. Instead of attempting to provide pregnant addicts with treatment alternatives, state and city attorneys pursued the prosecutorial route with extreme vigor. Because there were no statutes that specifically criminalized drug use during pregnancy (nor were there any that established criminal liability for maternal conduct resulting in prenatal injuries), prosecutors were forced to use existing laws in creative and often unprecedented ways (CRLP, 1993; Garrity-Rokous, 1994). Popular prosecutorial strategies included filing criminal charges for (a) child abuse and neglect, (b) involuntary manslaughter and homicide, and (c) use of controlled substances. By 1995, the American Civil Liberties Union (ACLU) estimated that 200 to 300 women had been prosecuted, generally under abuse and neglect statutes (ACLU Foundation, 1995).

Child Abuse and Neglect Statutes

The most common way of prosecuting women who use drugs during pregnancy is through abuse and neglect statutes. The first known prosecution using this approach was the 1977 case of *Reyes v. California,* wherein the defendant gave birth to twins—both of whom were addicted to heroin. The state attempted to prosecute Ms. Reyes under child endangerment laws, but the conviction was later overturned at the appellate level on grounds that the endangerment statute was never intended by the legislature to apply to fetuses.

In another significant case, *People v. Stewart* (1987), the defendant, Pamela Stewart of San Diego, was charged with criminal conduct following her inability to follow her doctor's advice regarding her pregnancy. Stewart was suffering from *placenta previa* (a condition in which the placenta is implanted in the lower portion of the uterus) and was ordered by her physician to avoid sexual intercourse and to immediately report for medical care in the event of any hemorrhaging. She engaged in vaginal intercourse, ingested amphetamines, and waited 12 hours before seeking medical care for her hemorrhaging. When her newborn was born brain damaged, tested positive for amphetamines, and died 6 weeks later, Ms. Stewart was charged and convicted of violating a California law that made it a misdemeanor for parents to "willfully omit, without legal excuse, to furnish necessary clothing, food, shelter or medical attendance, or other remedial care for his or her child" (*California Penal Code* 270, 1988). Ultimately, Ms. Stewart's conviction was overturned on the basis that the statute was never intended to apply to maternal conduct causing prenatal injury.

In both the *Reyes* and *Stewart* cases, as well as in the vast majority of subsequent abuse and neglect prosecutions, the central issues are, typically, (a) whether the fetus can be considered a "child" in the tradition of state child abuse-neglect laws and (b) whether prenatal conduct can be considered an appropriate criterion for the determination of abuse and neglect sanctions. In addition, in some jurisdictions, prosecutors must also demonstrate that abuse-neglect laws are intended to apply to maternal as well as third-party behavior. In addition to those in California, prosecutors in Colorado, Connecticut, Florida, Indiana, Michigan, Ohio, South Carolina, Texas, and Wyoming have used abuse-neglect laws to convict women who used drugs during their pregnancies (Garrity-Rokous, 1994). Most of these convictions have been successfully appealed, generally on the basis that child abuse laws are not intended to apply to fetuses or prenatal conduct. Nonetheless, written decisions in several cases that overturned the original convictions did not discourage states from pursuing such prosecutions (see *Ohio v. Gray*, 1992; *Welch v. Kentucky*, 1992). Instead, the high courts suggested that states pass legislation specifying that prenatal conduct is salient for abuse and neglect prosecutions, legislation that establishes the legal personhood of the fetus, or both.

Involuntary Manslaughter and Homicide

In a few state jurisdictions, prosecutors have charged mothers with homicide or manslaughter on grounds that the death of their newborn(s) was caused by prenatal drug use. In *Alaska v. Grubbs* (1989), for example, the defendant was charged with manslaughter after her newborn suffered a fatal heart attack believed to have been caused by prenatal cocaine exposure. Ms. Grubbs pleaded *nolo contendere* (no contest) to a lesser charge and was sentenced to 6 months in jail followed by probation. Similarly, in the case of *Illinois v. Green* (1989), prosecutors tried to charge a woman with manslaughter following the drug-related death of her newborn son. However, the grand jury refused to indict the defendant due to the inapplicability of the manslaughter statute and the prosecution's violation of the defendant's constitutional right to privacy.

Controlled Substances Statutes

Perhaps the most creative prosecutions of pregnant, drug-using women have been those engineered along the lines of drug statutes, particularly laws against trafficking and delivery of drugs to minors. Florida was the first state to successfully prosecute under this strategy in the well-known case of *Florida v. Johnson* (1989). Ms. Johnson was turned over to state prosecutors after hospital officials discovered that both of her children had positive toxicologies for cocaine following birth. She was subsequently convicted under a drug delivery statute on the basis that she had delivered cocaine to her newborn via the umbilical cord during the 60-second period after birth before the cord was cut. The infant's positive toxicology served as proof that she had delivered the drug. Prosecutors argued that the child could be considered a minor immediately following its birth (because Florida law does not recognize the legal personhood of a fetus). Ms. Johnson was subsequently sentenced to 15 years probation. In 1992, the Florida Supreme Court overturned her conviction on grounds that the statute was not intended to apply to cocaine delivery through the umbilical cord.

In a similar case, a Michigan appeals court overturned a drug delivery conviction on the basis that the statute was never intended to pertain to prenatal drug use (*Michigan v. Hardy*, 1991). The success of comparable prosecutions has been dependent on the court's interpretation of whether the fetus is a minor (according to legislative intent) and whether delivery statutes are intended to include transmission through umbilical cords.

Other Charges

Other criminal charges that have been unsuccessfully launched against pregnant drug users include contributing to the delinquency of a minor, causing the dependency of a child, drug possession, assault with a deadly weapon, vehicular homicide, and drug use. In the case of so-called pure use statutes, for example, prosecutors convict pregnant women of using an illegal substance based on the infant's positive toxicology screen. In so doing, prosecutors avoid having to demonstrate negligible harm to the fetus. Nonetheless, this type of prosecution appears to be limited to the state of Colorado because in other states a number of constitutional issues are raised around the (involuntary) testing of blood and the legal status of the fetus (Garrity-Rokous, 1994).

In addition, a number of judges have used their discretionary privilege to sanction women whom they suspect of prenatal substance use. Brenda Vaughn of Washington, DC, for example, was sentenced by the court to nearly 4 months in jail—an unusually long time for a first offender convicted of check forgery. Indeed, the typical sentence for this offense is probation, but Ms. Vaughn was a known cocaine user, and the judge felt that he had to protect her unborn child (*United States v. Vaughn,* 1988). In a more recent case, an Illinois trial judge sentenced a woman to 7 years in prison after charging her with violation of probation for failure to report to her probation officer and for using cocaine. The judge admitted to using this long sentence in an attempt to prevent the woman from becoming pregnant and giving birth to a cocaine-addicted child. The woman had recently given birth to a cocaine-addicted infant and had three other children in foster care with allegedly drug-related disabilities. An Illinois appellate court vacated this sentence indicating that the defendant's due process rights had been violated (*People of Illinois v. Bedenkop,* 1993).

Still other cases have targeted the prenatal ingestion of legal substances. In *Wyoming v. Pfannestiel* (1990), for example, officials charged a woman with child endangerment on grounds that her drinking might harm her unborn child. The case was ultimately dismissed on the basis that causality between alcohol consumption and harm had not been adequately established.

In general, these types of prosecutions have not withstood appellate review, largely because of the ambiguous legal status of the fetus and the departure of such prosecutions from the original intent of state legislatures. Nonetheless, criminal prosecutions have had profound consequences in the lives of many women, particularly those who lack the resources to challenge such claims. In 1992, the Reproductive Freedom Project of the ACLU initiated a study to track the cases of 167 women who had been arrested because of their allegedly criminal prenatal conduct. The study found that criminal prosecutions were launched in 24 states and the District of Columbia, although the vast majority were from South Carolina and Florida (Paltrow, 1992). In the majority of cases, women pleaded guilty or negotiated a plea to a lesser charge; in those cases where the defendant challenged the charge, it was nearly always dismissed. With the exception of California, the criminal prosecution of pregnant drug users ended with successful legal challenges.

More recently, the popularity of criminal prosecutions appears to have waned. During September 1994, for example, the Medical University of South Carolina announced that it would temporarily end its policy of forwarding names of pregnant women who test positive for cocaine to state prosecutors. The hospital was under pressure from the U.S. Department of Health and Human Services (DHHS) after the DHHS threatened to withdraw $18 million in federal research funding if the hospital continued to violate doctor-patient confidentiality and women's right to privacy. The old policy, known as the Interagency Policy on Management of Substance Abuse During Pregnancy or popularly referred to as the "crack baby program," required that doctors order drug tests if they suspected drug use (Jos, Marshall, & Perlnutter, 1995). If the test result was positive, the woman was ordered to enter drug treatment or be arrested. Under the policy, 42 pregnant women were arrested and charged with distributing cocaine to a minor. The new policy will require the hospital to petition the courts to have pregnant drug users committed (involuntarily) to drug treatment ("Hospital Gives Up," September 8, 1994, p. A18).

But in spite of these changes, some criminal prosecutions still occur. In Racine, Wisconsin, during early 1996, 35-year-old Deborah Zimmerman was charged with attempted murder after giving birth to a girl whose blood alcohol level was .199, nearly twice the threshold for a legal finding of intoxication. Moreover, the infant was smaller than normal and her forehead was somewhat flattened—a clear sign of fetal alcohol syndrome (Terry, 1996). Moreover, in *Whitner v. State* (1996), decided on July 15, 1996, the South Carolina Supreme Court ruled that a defendant who ingested crack during the third trimester of her pregnancy was properly prosecuted under the state's child abuse and endangerment statute. The appellate court emphasized that the statute's protection of persons under the age of 18 extended to a viable fetus.

Civil Actions

State actions via civil legal remedies have been more pervasive and considerably more successful than attempts at criminal prosecution (CRLP, 1993; Paltrow, 1992). This is not particularly surprising given that in criminal cases the burden of proof must be "beyond a reasonable doubt," whereas in civil cases the standard is a "preponderance of evidence." This grants states greater leeway in their justifications for intervention. Civil remedies have broadly included the use of child neglect statues, involuntary civil commitment, and tort actions.

Child Neglect Statutes

Unlike criminal findings of abuse and neglect, civil neglect statutes allow social welfare agencies (typically, child welfare organizations) to intervene and assume responsibility for care of children whose parents are under investigation for potential parental misconduct. Rather than punishment-oriented in the sense that the parent is sanctioned or penalized (although it could be argued that the loss of one's child or children constitutes a more significant penalty than incarceration), neglect statutes are deemed forward looking in that they allow intervention on the basis of both present harm and predicted future harm (Garrity-Rokous, 1994). The central issue in most neglect interventions is the question of whether a positive toxicology screen at birth is sufficient to establish neglect and, ultimately, revoke parental custody. Also at issue is whether a mother's prenatal drug use (or conduct in general) can be used to establish a finding of future harm.

With regard to positive toxicology screens at birth, in the 1985 case of *In the Matter of Danielle Smith*, a New York court found evidence of neglect on the basis of the mother's prenatal alcohol use. The state's neglect statute requires a finding of either actual harm or imminent future harm. Although the court could not establish that fetal harm had indeed occurred, it did find that the mother's behavior was sufficiently detrimental to demonstrate imminent future harm. Similarly, in another New York case (*In the Matter of Stefenal, Tyesha C.*, 1990), the court found that a positive toxicology screen for cocaine at birth was enough to establish harm and evidence of neglect. This court, like its predecessor, held that New York neglect statutes were applicable to maternal prenatal conduct.

The Supreme Court of Connecticut's decision in the case of *In re Valerie D.* (1992) served as the basis for answering the second question related to civil intervention—can prenatal drug use serve as a sufficient basis for the revocation of custody? In its original verdict, the court used the same reasoning as earlier New York cases to support a finding of future harm and the termination of parental rights. In this case, an infant was born with evidence of cocaine in her bloodstream. The state filed petitions of neglect and custody termination immediately, and then 70 days after assuming custody of the child, the state also charged the mother with abandonment. The local court's reasoning in the case was that a single positive toxicology at birth was sufficient evidence of parental unfitness and an accurate predictor of future harm to the child. The case was overturned by the state Supreme Court, however, on the basis that the state's neglect statute had been misinterpreted by the lower court. The appellate court held that the legislature had never intended for parental rights to be terminated on the basis of prenatal conduct, thereby disallowing the results of a single drug test to serve as the sole basis for a judgment of neglect.

It is important to note that although the Connecticut Supreme Court overturned the lower court decision, the written opinion in the case did not preclude that state or any others from approving legislation that would specifically define prenatal drug use as constitutive of abuse and neglect. Indeed, other states have continued to use positive toxicologies to establish neglect and proceed with civil intervention cases (Garrity-Rokous, 1994).

Emerging from the area of family law are two influential cases, both of which ruled that a child has a "right" to be born with a "sound mind and body" (Madden, 1993). The first was a Michigan case, *In re Baby X* (1980), which involved a child who exhibited drug withdrawal symptoms at birth. A probate court determined the newborn's poor health was sufficient evidence of neglect and validated the termination of parental custody rights. On appeal, the mother argued that prenatal conduct cannot serve as grounds for a finding of neglect. The court ruled that prenatal conduct is material and relevant to investigations of neglect given that (a) children have a right to be born with a sound mind and body and (b) neglect proceedings can use parental treatment of one child to serve as evidence in a neglect case filed on behalf of a different child (thereby establishing that past conduct is relevant in determining future harm).

In the Ohio case of *In re Ruiz* (1986), the court reiterated the right of the child to be born with a sound mind and body. In this case, the child was born addicted to heroin. The court held that this was constitutive of abuse and that a viable fetus could be considered a child under the rubric of child endangerment statutes.

Involuntary Civil Commitment

Civil commitment refers to state intervention that places individuals in some type of inpatient facility against their will after the state has demonstrated that they are dangerous or unable to meet their most basic needs or both. This type of intervention has been widely applied to substance abusers; indeed, 33 states specifically allow involuntary commitment for persons addicted to drugs (Garcia & Segalman, 1991). In these cases, the state must establish that the pregnant drug user is dangerous to herself and *others,* thus raising the issue of the legal status of a fetus.

At present, only Minnesota has been able to successfully include pregnant women in statutes allowing for commitment of substance abusers (Garrity-Rokous, 1994). As such, health care workers are required to report women they suspect of prenatal drug use. If the woman refuses treatment services, a local welfare agency must petition for involuntary commitment (the commitment itself may last up to 6 months and may be renewed).

The case of *In re Steven S.* (1981) is important in this regard even though it did not involve charges of prenatal drug use. In this case, a pregnant woman who was believed to have a mental disorder (though not diagnosed) was ordered into state custody to protect her fetus under California's child neglect statute. An appeals court overturned the decision on the basis that the juvenile court lacked jurisdiction and that the fetus was not a legal person under the state's abuse statute. However, the court maintained that the commitment could have legally proceeded from the state's civil commitment statute.

Tort Actions

Tort actions are intended to deter prenatal substance abuse by holding women accountable for the economic costs associated with the birth of drug-exposed infants. Tort actions require that someone (usually other family members) bring an action on behalf of the fetus (Keyes, 1992). The most important case involving tort action in this behalf was based on the ingestion of a legal substance—tetracycline.

In *Grodin v. Grodin* (1981), the mother admitted using prescribed tetracycline during her pregnancy, although she discontinued its use when she learned she was pregnant. Her child was born with discolored teeth, and the father sued her for monetary damages on behalf of the child. In Michigan, any person (including parents) who causes prenatal injury through negligence can be held liable. In this case, the court ruled that the mother could be held liable as determined by a judge or jury (Keyes, 1992).

In general, civil abuse and custody proceedings occur even more frequently than criminal prosecutions. Only eight states currently mandate that hospital staff report a newborn's positive toxicology as evidence of child abuse or neglect, although hundreds of women around the nation have had their children removed from their custody on the basis of alleged drug or alcohol use during pregnancy (CRLP, 1993).

Constitutional Issues

Punitive state intervention with regard to prenatal substance abuse raises a number of significant legal questions—roughly divided into constitutional issues and statutory limitations. Nearly all the cases that have gone to appellate courts have been challenged on the basis of legislative intent. State courts have been hesitant to address the constitutional issues implicated in the prosecution of prenatal conduct and have decided the majority according to whether or not the intervention could reasonably fall within the boundaries set by state legislatures (including the legal status of the fetus in the state's legislative history). Primarily, issues raised against punitive intervention center around the Fourteenth Amendment, rights of privacy, and more narrowly implicate Fourth and Eighth Amendment rights.

Fourteenth Amendment

At the center of the constitutional controversy surrounding state intervention in the lives of pregnant drug users and their fetuses are such Fourteenth Amendment issues as due process, liberty, and equal protection. As stated in the Fourteenth Amendment, "nor shall any State deprive any person of . . . liberty . . . without due process of law; nor deny any person within its jurisdiction the equal protection of the laws."

Due Process

The due process clause asserts, in effect, that the state must have a clearly defined objective related to public health, safety, or welfare to justify its intervention in the lives of citizens (Andrews & Patterson, 1995). In demonstrating its interest in a particular matter (e.g., drug use among pregnant women), the state must show that the planned intervention (i.e., criminal prosecution) is related to accomplishing its goal (i.e., protecting the fetus from negative effects associated with certain substances) and that there is a reasonable degree of certainty that the intervention will work toward accomplishing this goal. In addition, the state must show that the benefits to be gained from the intervention will outweigh the costs of that intervention to individual rights. If fundamental rights such as liberty, privacy, or bodily integrity are to be affected, the state must demonstrate that the intervention is reasonable (e.g., it can be expected to accomplish the goal), narrowly constructed, and that there is no less intrusive way to accomplish the goal (Andrews & Patterson, 1995; Garrity-Rokous, 1994).

State intervention in the lives of pregnant substance users has raised a number of due process issues.

Criminal Prosecution. Can prosecution be reasonably expected to either deter women from using drugs during their pregnancies or protect the fetus from immediate harm caused by substance use? Has the state sufficiently established that prenatal drug use is a criminal act and therefore provided adequate notification to persons affected? Does criminal prosecution violate the fundamental rights of the mother, and if so, can this form of intervention be justified on the basis that it contributes to a greater good?

Civil Intervention. It has been argued that the right to raise one's child is a fundamental right that falls within past Supreme Court decisions regarding parental authority and reproductive privacy, thereby calling into question the state's practice of terminating custody rights of women who used drugs during their pregnancies. Similarly, involuntary commitment raises questions regarding mothers' fundamental rights (Andrews & Patterson, 1995).

Physician Disclosure. Laws requiring that physicians disclose the results of toxicologies to law enforcement agents or allow medical records to be used in prosecutions, or both, potentially violate women's rights to privacy and freedom of association (Andrews & Patterson, 1995; Chavkin, 1990; Farr, 1995). Furthermore, it could be argued that physicians who forward patient records to law enforcement function as law enforcement agents themselves. As such, they are required to obtain informed consent from their patients before engaging in any kind of testing that could result in criminal prosecution. Failure to obtain informed consent would potentially violate Fourth Amendment protection against illegal search and seizure (Chavkin, 1990).

Collection of Evidence. The collection of evidence against the mother in most civil and criminal cases is also problematic because it is often taken without her consent or knowledge. Most criminal and civil cases to date have been based on blood tests performed on the newborn. This raises serious questions regarding the right of health care workers to perform tests intended for state intervention on persons who do not have the capacity to make an informed choice and raises issues about parental consent and authority (Farr, 1995).

Clearly, it appears difficult to justify criminal prosecutions of any kind given the conditions of the due process requirement. It appears that prosecution neither deters drug-using women from becoming pregnant (though it may encourage abortions or avoidance of pre-natal care) nor does it deter them from using drugs. A number of scholars have argued that criminal prosecutions are misguided social policies because they fail to acknowledge the enduring nature of addiction (Watkins & Watkins, 1992). Furthermore, this type of intervention does little to protect the fetus, because many women find themselves in correctional facilities that are notorious for their lack of adequate obstetric care, dietary resources, and abundance of illegal drugs (King, 1992; Watkins & Watkins, 1992). Last, it may also be noted that criminal prosecutions and the burden they place on the fundamental rights of pregnant women cannot adequately be justified by looking to the rights of the fetus. As numerous Supreme Court decisions have attested (most notably *Roe v. Wade* in 1973), the fetus is not entitled to the same rights as persons under the framework of the Constitution nor can fetuses be considered persons under the Court's interpretation of the concept (Andrews & Patter-son, 1995; CRLP, 1993).

A secondary issue raised within the scope of the due process clause involves the right of citizens to be informed of conduct that is considered criminal. It has been argued that the attempts of some

states to manipulate existing statutes (e.g., laws criminalizing delivery of drugs to minors) in order to prosecute pregnant, drug-using
women are unconstitutional because the defendant had no previous
awareness that her conduct was illegal (Farr, 1995). Indeed, the very
intent of the due process clause is to prevent prosecutors from
inventing new crimes or from interpreting statutes in unintended
and ambiguous ways (Garrity-Rokous, 1994). Because no statutes
currently exist to criminalize drug use among pregnant women, the
argument is that states have failed to provide fair notice of criminal
conduct. Use of preexisting statutes to criminalize heretofore unregulated behavior, as such, is unconstitutional (Farr, 1995).

Equal Protection

According to the Fourteenth Amendment, the state must also
demonstrate that its intervention is equitable—that is, that the law
will be applied to all persons who are similarly situated. If the
category of persons is "pregnant, drug-using women," the state must
show that this category is relevant to the intervention and appropriate. Some have argued that to demonstrate the category's relevance,
it must be shown that pregnant drug users as a whole generate a
known harm (Andrews & Patterson, 1995). There is no consensus
in the medical research community as to the harm caused by prenatal
drug use (particularly because it appears associated with other
factors such as malnutrition and inadequate prenatal care). Moreover, a number of women who have used drugs during their pregnancies have given birth to healthy infants, whereas others have
babies with compounded health problems (Hawk, 1994; Maher,
1990). As such, "pregnant, drug-using women" does not appear to
be a category that sufficiently establishes a causal relationship between the criminal act (prenatal drug use) and the resulting injury
(harm to the fetus).[1]

Furthermore, this category must be applied fairly; that is, it must
not discriminate among members who are similarly situated. A
number of sources, however, have suggested that state intervention
is overwhelmingly applied to low-income, minority women (Chasnoff,
Landress, & Barrett, 1990; Paltrow, 1992). For example, a study
conducted in Pinellas County, Florida, found that pregnant African
American women who use drugs and alcohol during their pregnancies are 10 times more likely to be reported to authorities than white
women, even though rates of prenatal drug use among black and
white women are roughly equal (Chasnoff et al., 1990). Similarly, a

survey of known criminal cases undertaken by the ACLU revealed that 70% of those forwarded for prosecution involved minority defendants (CRLP, 1993). Discriminatory treatment often occurs because prosecutors and other state agents must rely on health care workers to forward evidence of prenatal drug use. Because drug testing of mother and infant is left to the discretion of health care workers in most jurisdictions, it is not surprising that testing is most frequently undertaken in urban hospitals and among minority women (CRLP, 1993; Smith & Dabiri, 1991). Furthermore, many investigations of prenatal drug exposure are based on negative effects associated with crack cocaine and other illegal drugs. Considerably less attention has focused on the ingestion of legal substances, such as alcohol, tranquilizers, and other prescription medications that are more frequently used by middle-class women.

Rights to Privacy

The argument has been made that prenatal drug abuse laws and criminal prosecutions potentially intrude on two aspects of a woman's right to privacy (Keyes, 1992). The first involves the right to privacy regarding reproductive decisions as elaborated in *Griswold v. Connecticut* (1965) and implied in the penumbras of the First, Third, Fourth, Fifth, and Ninth Amendments to the Constitution. The second involves a woman's right to bodily integrity, established in a number of court decisions relating to the Fourth Amendment. The point is that prenatal substance abuse laws and prosecutions potentially violate these rights when they prohibit pregnant women from engaging in conduct they did prior to pregnancy, when they impose harsher penalties on women substance abusers who are pregnant, or both. Under proposed prenatal abuse laws, a woman who wants to drink alcohol cannot choose to be pregnant. This would violate fundamental rights to privacy and should fall under the rubric of strict scrutiny standards, although the Supreme Court has been unwilling to apply strict scrutiny to a number of recent cases involving reproductive privacy (Keyes, 1992). Subsequently, although a constitutional challenge may be launched against prenatal abuse laws, it is doubtful that such laws will be nullified on the basis of a woman's right to privacy given the Court's willingness to abandon the viability test as the starting point for compelling state interest in the life of the fetus (see *Webster v. Reproductive Health Services,* 1989).

Eighth Amendment

Some scholars, most notably ACLU representatives, have also argued that the criminal prosecution of pregnant, drug-using women raises questions regarding the Eighth Amendment ban against cruel and unusual punishment. One position, for example, holds that the efforts to prosecute maternal fetal abuse of any kind amount to criminalization of pregnancy itself, because "no woman can provide the perfect womb" (Paltrow, 1992). Whether or not fetal abuse cases criminalize pregnancy, there does appear to be some merit in the claim that prosecuting women for prenatal conduct is constitutive of cruel and unusual punishment. In *Robinson v. California* (1962), the Supreme Court nullified a state statute that made it a crime to be addicted to drugs. The court's decision was based on medical knowledge that characterized addiction to alcohol and drugs as a disease. The Court concluded that criminalizing a medical condition or social status constituted cruel and unusual punishment. Subsequently, some scholars have argued that prosecutions of drug-using, pregnant women amount to nothing more than criminalization of a condition (Farr, 1995; Watkins & Watkins, 1992). This appears particularly evident in cases wherein a pregnant woman is prosecuted for alcohol use (a legal behavior) during her pregnancy (see *Wyoming v. Pfannestiel*, 1990)—in effect, she is being prosecuted for the condition or status of being pregnant. In addition, several researchers have noted that prosecution of pregnant substance abusers is based on the faulty assumption that addicts have the capacity to terminate their drug habits at will (Farr, 1995; Hawk, 1994; Madden, 1993). These scholars argue that addiction clouds the capacity of pregnant women to terminate drug use; as such, efforts to punish these women for failing to overcome addiction are violative of the Eighth Amendment.

Cocaine Use and Fetal Rights

An issue often linked to discussions of drug use during pregnancy is the intensifying debate over so-called fetal rights. Although the notion of fetal rights has received considerable attention in recent years, the movement has a history spanning almost three decades (Lieb & Sterk-Elifson, 1995; Watkins & Watkins, 1992). The emergence of fetal rights as a topic for social and legal debate has been attributed to the civil rights movement of the 1960s. Civil rights activists were able to secure legal recognition for people who had traditionally been denied their rights under the law, and some segments of society wished to extend this protection to fetuses, whom they considered to be among the most dispossessed of groups (Watkins & Watkins, 1992).

Since its inception, the fetal rights movement has maintained that the fetus is a person, that the fetus possesses an existence that is separate from that of its mother, and that this existence should be legally acknowledged. Protective statutes for full-term, viable fetuses have been in existence since the 1961 court decision in *Hoener v. Bertinato* (Bowes & Selgestad, 1981). However, the 1960s saw no successful prosecutions with respect to fetal rights violations, perhaps because the benefits of parenthood were thought to outweigh any damages (Weinstein, 1983).

The fetal rights movement began to gain a stronger foothold throughout the nation during the early 1970s. The 1973 decision rendered in *Roe v. Wade* included language that asserted the state's compelling interest in the life of an unborn fetus (Dal Pazzo & Marsh, 1987). Many interested parties viewed this judgment as recognition of the separate interest of the fetus, which heretofore had not been acknowledged. Conventional medical opinion had regarded the mother and fetus as a unit, with no existence of the fetus apart from that of the mother. Subsequent to *Roe v. Wade,* a 1977 Rhode Island court ruled that a child was legally entitled to begin life with a sound mind and body, thus validating the right of a fetus to sue for damages (Weinstein, 1983).

Going further, some proponents of fetal rights argue that once abortion is no longer an option in the pregnancy (either as a result of statutory prohibitions or a woman's choice not to abort), the court should favor the interests of the fetus over those of its mother (Tomkins & Kepfield, 1992). Fetal rights proponents argue that fetuses have a fundamental right to be born with a sound mind and body. This latter point served as the basis for decisions favoring the fetus in *In re Baby X* (1980), *Grodin v. Grodin* (1980), and *In re Ruiz* (1986). Tomkins and Kepfield (1992) argue that even in the *Roe* case, the Court recognized the state's interests in upholding the rights of the fetus at the point of viability. In this case, the Court noted that the woman and her fetus have separate and distinct rights that must be balanced throughout the duration of the pregnancy. During the first trimester, the woman's rights to reproductive privacy take precedence over any interests of the fetus. At the point of viability, however, the balance shifts in favor of the fetus and legitimates the state's protection of fetal rights (through the regulation of abortion) unless the mother's life or health is in jeopardy.

The decision in *Roe v. Wade*, among others (see *Webster v. Reproductive Health Services*, 1989), establishes the legitimacy of the state's interest in protecting the rights of the fetus. As such, intervention in the form of criminal prosecution or civil proceedings is entirely justified, particularly in cases of prenatal drug use that occurs after the point of viability. However, those who favor this type of state intervention often fail to address the issue of harm beyond citing earlier studies attesting to the damaging effects of cocaine or alcohol on fetal development nor do they mention the inequity that has characterized the vast majority of criminal prosecutions and termination of custody proceedings. Rather, they take harm as a given and argue that child abuse statutes are particularly suited to state intervention because drug use is constitutive of abuse that places a child in imminent harm (Tomkins & Kepfield, 1992).

The decisions in the *Roe* and *Webster* cases laid the foundation for court-mandated obstetric interventions to be sanctioned in many areas of the country. Court-ordered nontherapeutic cesarean sections (see *In re AC 573 A.2d 1235*), hospital detentions, and intrauterine transfusions have been imposed on substance-abusing women, terminally ill women, and still others with strong religious objections to medical intervention (Rosner et al., 1989). Although the American College of Obstetricians and Gynecologists issued a statement in 1987 that court-mandated treatment is inadvisable and may eventually result in the criminalization of noncompliance with medical regimens (Justin & Rosner, 1989), state courts and legislatures continue to grant rights to fetuses that have heretofore been reserved for persons (Rosner et al., 1989).

As noted earlier, in response to the barrage of crack baby stories that appeared in the media throughout the late 1980s and early 1990s, several states tried to adapt existing criminal child neglect and abuse legislation to include the unborn (Peak & Del Papa, 1993), thus allowing for the prosecution of the mothers. Several cases were unsuccessfully prosecuted (*People v. Morabito*, 1992; *Ohio v. Gray*, 1992; *State v. Andrews*, 1989) when the courts concluded that a fetus did not constitute a child within the child endangerment statutes (Peak & Del Papa, 1993). The decision in *People v. Morabito* further emphasized that it was the responsibility of the legislature to "criminalize the ingestion of cocaine during pregnancy when such ingestion results in harm to the subsequently born child (Peak &

Del Papa, 1993, p. 252). So far, no state has created legislation to impose additional criminal penalties on pregnant drug users (Lieb & Sterk-Elifson, 1995). One major obstacle to the implementation of such legislation may be the difficulty encountered in trying to establish a connection between the mother's drug use and harm to the fetus (Watkins & Watkins, 1992). As stated by Mariner, Glantz, and Annas (1990),

> As a practical matter, it seems almost impossible to satisfy the standard of proof of causation in a criminal prosecution, given the complexity of fetal development. . . . The further assumption is needed that drug use alone or fetal harm alone are themselves independent forms of culpable behavior. If drug use alone is not a crime, then what is being punished is the status of being pregnant. (p. 34)

Postscript

As the use of cocaine escalated during the 1980s, one of the many new drug control strategies was the notion of *user accountability*. User accountability was based on the idea that if there were no drug users, there would be no drug problems and that users were responsible for creating the demand that made trafficking a lucrative criminal enterprise (Inciardi, 1992). User accountability brought forth many new laws calling for mandatory penalties for those found in possession of even small amounts of illegal drugs. The same ethos also stimulated the movement toward prosecuting pregnant addicts.

A second influence was the antiabortion movement. Pro-life and fetal rights advocates were insisting that the state must intervene in cases of prenatal drug abuse to ensure proper medical care for both mother and child. More important, however, the issue of prenatal drug use was amenable to the pro-life agenda to chip away at the 1973 decision in *Roe v. Wade*, which granted women the right to an abortion and limited fetal rights (McGinnis, 1990). As such, the social and political environments were ready for state intervention.

Not surprisingly, those in favor of punitive approaches to the problem of prenatal drug abuse tend to be conservative politicians, prosecutors in a few states, and persons interested in expanding fetal rights—including pro-life activists. Their interests can generally be categorized as belonging primarily to (a) a deterrence philosophy of criminal punishment and (b) a belief in the government's right to protect the interests of the fetus over and against any rights possessed by the mother.

Persons belonging to the deterrence school argue that prenatal drug exposure is a serious crime that presents a potentially life-threatening situation for the fetus and incurs significant financial costs that are often shouldered by the taxpayer (Keyes, 1992). They contend that drug use is a crime from which pregnant women should not be exempt simply as a result of carrying an unborn child. To prevent prenatal drug use and protect the health and well-being of the fetus, proponents argue that women should be fully prosecuted. In sum, proponents believe punishment would serve to deter the mother's motivation to engage in future drug use, encourage her to seek drug treatment she may otherwise have avoided, and demonstrate to other women that their illicit behavior will involve significant costs to their freedom, finances, or both (Condon, 1995).

It is interesting that there appears to be no empirical evidence supporting the position of deterrence advocates. Indeed, because many of these advocates are prosecutors and activists, they generally present their position in popular news magazines, citing anecdotal information as proof of the effectiveness of criminal prosecution. One of the most visible deterrence advocates is South Carolina Attorney General Charles Molony Condon. He suggests that an evaluative study of South Carolina's perinatal abuse policy is demonstrative of its success. As mentioned earlier, South Carolina instituted the crack-baby program that forced pregnant mothers who tested positive for cocaine to either enter treatment or face arrest and possible conviction on drug delivery charges. Citing the high cost of hospital treatment and the moral decay of substance-abusing mothers, Condon concluded that the crack-baby program was a phenomenal success. The state-commissioned study reported that before the policy took effect, about 24 pregnant women a month tested positive for cocaine, and virtually none were willing to voluntarily seek treatment. In 1989, following the introduction of the new policy, the number of pregnant women testing positive for cocaine decreased to only 5 or 6 per month, and there was no evidence that women were deterred from seeking prenatal treatment (Condon, 1995). Condon's program was later shut down by the DHHS following reports that it targeted lower-class, minority women (testing occurred in urban hospitals and at the discretion of the health care provider) and was overly coercive.

Advocates of fetal rights, whereas often in agreement with deterrence philosophy, have a motive in their support of state intervention—expanding the rights of the fetus (particularly in a direction that would ultimately overturn the *Roe* decision and make all abortions illegal). Advocates of this movement are less interested in examining the effects of punitive interventions on pregnant women than they are in establishing the harm the fetus incurs as a result of prenatal drug exposure. Besharov (1989), among others, cited early medical reports of the effects of cocaine on the fetus and reproduced estimates of the ever-growing numbers of fetuses exposed to hazardous substances. Fetal rights advocates also view mother and fetus as competitors (rather than as interdependent) and adopt a moral view of the crack mother as selfish, irresponsible, cruel, and neglectful (see Besharov, 1989, 1990; Condon, 1995). Thus, punitive action is particularly justified in light of the cruelty implicated in exposing the fetus to the toxic effects of crack cocaine.

There have been a number of critiques raised against punitive intervention by a variety of individuals and interest groups. Among those who generally oppose criminal sanctions are physicians (and pediatricians in particular), child welfare and social service workers, social science researchers, feminists, liberal politicians, addictions counselors, and many legal advocates (CRLP, 1993).

One of the most often cited criticisms of punitive intervention is that it will serve to deter pregnant women from seeking treatment for fear they will be prosecuted or will have their babies taken away from them (Hawk, 1994; Keyes, 1992). Although it does not appear that any rigorous empirical investigations have been undertaken to support this claim, there is an increasing body of anecdotal evidence that indicates that drug-using mothers are avoiding treatment and prenatal programs (Larson, 1991). Indeed, this may have been the case in South Carolina's crack-baby program where Condon cites a dramatic drop in the numbers of pregnant women testing positive for cocaine (Condon, 1995). Also, critics fear that punitive sanctions will prevent pregnant women from revealing to health care workers their drug use and other information that would be vital to tailoring prenatal treatment to meet the special needs of the woman and her baby (Watkins & Watkins, 1992).

In addition, negative sanctions, such as incarceration or fines, do little to prevent or even inhibit drug use during or after pregnancy. It has been established empirically that illegal drugs are generally available in prison (Inciardi, 1996) and that prisons often lack the resources to provide drug treatment, obstetric care, and adequate dietary requirements for pregnant women. In this scenario, punitive sanctions may do more harm to the fetus than good (Keyes, 1992). Furthermore, incarceration serves to disrupt families and contributes to the problem of boarder babies—that is, newborns who are forced to remain in hospitals for months because of criminal or civil litigation pending against their mothers (Farr, 1995).

Another anticipated consequence of punitive intervention is the "slippery slope" hypothesis. Here, critics argue that criminalizing drug use during pregnancy will necessarily lead to criminalization of legal behaviors, such as alcohol or tobacco use, that also appear to have negative effects on fetal development (Paltrow, 1992). Furthermore, because no woman can provide the perfect womb, prosecution for prenatal drug use may open the door to prosecuting women for any variety of activities during their pregnancies and may subject pregnant women to any number of regulations that deprive them of basic constitutional rights (King, 1992; Paltrow, 1992). The Nevada Supreme Court illustrates this dilemma in its ruling that Nevada's child endangerment statute does not apply to a pregnant woman's ingestion of illegal drugs:

> To hold otherwise would ascribe to the legislature the intent to criminalize the conduct of women who ingest any substance that has the potential to harm a fetus. This would open the floodgates to prosecution of pregnant women who ingest such things as alcohol, nicotine, and a range of miscellaneous, otherwise legal, toxins. (*Nevada v. Encoe,* 1994)

The U.S. Supreme Court has ruled that addiction is an illness and not willful, criminal behavior. The American Medical Association has recommended a medical rather than a punitive approach to maternal drug use. Those in favor of punitive approaches generally assume that pregnant women willfully and criminally choose to hurt their fetus through the ingestion of damaging substances. Little empirical research exists to support these claims. Indeed, one study of drug-using mothers reveals that the mothers are motivated to seek help for their drug use precisely because they do not want to harm their children (Maher, 1990). Unfortunately, the women who are motivated to seek help overcoming their substance use are often confronted by the grim reality that little help is available to them. An interesting footnote to the 1987 case of *Florida v. Johnson* (the mother who was charged with delivery of cocaine to a minor through her umbilical cord) is that Jennifer Johnson, apparently motivated by concern for the health of her future child, had tried to get treatment for her drug addiction but was turned away because she was pregnant (Golden, 1991). Ms. Johnson was, ironically, later ordered to complete drug treatment as part of her sentencing. A 1989 survey of 54 drug treatment programs in New York City (representing 95% of the programs citywide) found that 54% refused to treat pregnant women, 67% denied treatment to pregnant women on Medicaid, and 87% denied treatment to Medicaid recipients addicted to crack (Chavkin, 1990; see also Breitbart, Chavkin, & Wise, 1994).

It appears urgent that public policy toward prenatal substance abuse move in the direction of providing necessary rehabilitative and social welfare services. Gains made by punitive intervention strategies are limited at best and frequently exacerbate the tendency among substance users to avoid seeking prenatal care, thereby causing greater harm to infants at risk. Indeed, a number of states have begun to investigate rehabilitative, as opposed to punitive, intervention strategies. California, Connecticut, the District of Columbia, Florida, Illinois, Kentucky, Minnesota, Missouri, and Wisconsin, among others, have expanded drug treatment services to accommodate pregnant clients. Numerous other states have appointed commissions in recent years to investigate the problem of prenatal drug use and provide recommendations for sound public policy.

States must also continue to educate women and the general public about pregnancy and substance abuse. There are still many misperceptions about the effects of different substances on the fetus. The incorrect perception that the placenta protects the fetus to varying degrees throughout a woman's pregnancy continues to exist. For example, women commonly believe that drugs can harm the fetus only in the beginning of a pregnancy. In one survey, it was found that 90% of women knew that alcohol could harm the fetus during the first trimester, whereas only 46.8% and 44.2% of women knew that there were risks in the second and third trimesters (Castelli, 1993). Education can clear up these misperceptions and provide new information to those populations at risk and to the hidden populations—the middle-class and upper-class drug users who can more easily escape the consequences of their drug use.

Last, the media's focus on crack cocaine has in fact done women and society a disservice. In overrepresenting crack as a demon drug that causes great damage to the fetus, the harmful effects of alcohol and tobacco, affecting many more lives and perhaps having a greater detrimental effect on the fetus than does cocaine, have been greatly downplayed. The mean-spirited and frenzied nature of media forecasting regarding the crack baby generation has provided little, if any, accurate information about prenatal substance abuse and has unduly guided public policy toward increasingly punitive measures that have been found to be not only unconstitutional, but highly ineffective.

Note

1. Indeed, it is not even clear that women should be solely responsible for the health of the fetus. One study of cocaine-using fathers found that cocaine may bind to human sperm, where it is then transported into the ovum, potentially leading to the abnormal development of the offspring (Yazigi, Odem, & Polakoski, 1991).

Epilogue

Overall, although there is no consensus as to the effects of cocaine on the infant and child, it is generally agreed by both the medical and research communities that cocaine has at least the potential to be harmful to the mother and her growing fetus. Moreover, it is generally agreed that some fetuses who are exposed to cocaine will be adversely affected but that the extent of the damage was likely overstated in the beginning. Indeed, much research has shown that most cocaine-exposed infants are either unaffected by or overcome their exposure.

At the same time, it is apparent that researchers and clinicians are not completely sure what to look for in terms of the effects of cocaine. It may be the case that because we have not yet adequately measured problems, we have only begun to uncover the detrimental effects of this drug. There is a considerable need for the development of mechanisms designed for the observation of cocaine-exposed infants and their caregivers to describe characteristics worthy of further study (Barton, Harrigan, & Tse, 1995).

The following quote made by prominent researchers of cocaine-exposed infants clearly sums up what is known (and not known) about cocaine's effects on the fetus, the newborn, and the child:

Like prematurity, drug exposure can be viewed as another *potential* insult or injury to the developing fetus. We do not know if and how drugs affect the fetus; we do not know the effects of polydrug use; we do not know the effects of timing, dosage, and frequency of use. In some infants there may be true injury, in others there may be any degree of insult and many infants may escape unscathed. It is also possible that there are effects that we simply do not know how to measure or effects that are not manifest until the child is older. Also, drug effects will interact with other prenatal factors such as poor nutrition or illness that may also potentially compromise the infant (Lester & Tronick, 1994, p. 116).

Research to date has generally indicated that the majority of cocaine-exposed infants are born without pervasive physical or neurobehavioral impairments and show normal development in later infancy. However, large-scale studies of the subsequent development of cocaine-exposed children have only recently begun—how these children will fare over time remains uncertain (Hawley et al., 1995).

As the field enters the second generation of research on cocaine-exposed infants, perhaps most important, a better understanding of the actual problem has been established. Lester and Tronick (1994) explain that the two main issues that have emerged over 10 years of research on prenatal exposure to cocaine are that (a) cocaine use is really polydrug use and (b) environment or lifestyle, which includes both psychological and social factors, plays a significant role in developmental outcome.

Although findings from early research of infants exposed prenatally to cocaine may have exaggerated the severity of the situation in the beginning, this does not mean that the potential adverse effects of cocaine on the exposed fetus should be ignored. Many infants do appear to escape from cocaine unharmed, but others may experience subtle problems later in life. At this point, because there is no solid understanding about the effects of cocaine on the fetus, the unborn child should be viewed as having the potential to experience adverse effects from prenatal cocaine exposure.

Court Cases

Alaska v. Grubbs, No. 4FA S89 415 Criminal (Sup. Ct. August 25, 1989).
California Penal Code 270 (1988).
Dietrich v. Inhabitants of Northampton, 138 Mass. 14, 52 Am. Rep. 242 (1884).
Florida v. Johnson, No. 89-1765 [Cir. Ct., July 13, 1989].
Griswold v. Connecticut, 381 U.S. 479 (1965).
Grodin v. Grodin, 102 Mich. 396, 301 N.W.2d 869 (1980).
Hoener v. Bertinato, 67 N.J. Sup. 517 171A 2d 140, 1961.
In re AC 573 A.2d 1235.
In re Baby X, 97 Mich. App. 111, 293 N.W.2d 736 (1980).
In re Ruiz, 27 Ohio Misc. 2d 31, 32 (Ct. of Common Pleas 1986).
In re Steven S., 126 Cal. App. 3d 23, 178 Cal. Rptr. 525 (1981).
In re Valerie D., 3 223 Conn. 492 (1992).
In the Matter of Danielle Smith, 128 Misc. 2d 976, 492 N.Y.S. 2d 331 (1985).
In the Matter of Stefenal, Tyesha C., 556 N.Y.S.2d 280 (App. Div. 1990).
Johnson v. Florida, 602 So.2d 1288 (Fla. 1992).
Michigan v. Hardy, 469 N.W.2d 50 (188 Mich. App. 305, 1991).
Nevada v. Encoe, Nev SupCt, No. 24888 (11/30/94).
Ohio v. Gray, 584 N.E. 2d 710 (Ohio 1992).
People of Illinois v. Bedenkop, Ill AppCt, 1stDist, No. 1-92-0604 (8/13/93).
People of Illinois v. Green, No. 88-CM-8256 (Cir. Ct. filed May 8, 1989).
People v. Morabito, 580 N.Y.S.2d 843 (1992).
People v. Stewart, No. M 508197 (San Diego Mun. Ct., Feb. 23, 1987).
Reyes v. California, 75 Cal. App3d. 214 (1977).
Robinson v. California, 370 US 660, 8 L ed 2d 758, 82 S Ct 1417 [No 554].
Roe v. Wade, 410 U.S. 113 (1973).

State v. Andrews, Family Court of Stark County, Ohio (19 June 1989).
United States v. Vaughn, No. F-2172-88B (D.C. Super. Ct. August 23, 1988).
Webster v. Reproductive Health Services, 492 U.S. 490 (1989).
Welch v. Kentucky, No 90-CA-1189-MR (Ky. Ct. App. Feb. 7, 1992).
Whitner v. State, 59 CrL 1377 (1996).
Wyoming v. Pfannestiel, No. 1-90-8CR (Co. Ct. of Laramie, Wyoming, Feb. 1, 1990).

References

Agar, M. (1973). *Ripping and running: A formal ethnography of urban heroin addicts.* New York: Seminar Press.

American Civil Liberties Union Foundation. (1995). *Criminal prosecutions against pregnant women.* New York: Center for Reproductive Law and Policy.

Andrews, A. B., & Patterson, E. (1995). Searching for solutions to alcohol and other drug abuse during pregnancy: Ethics, values, and constitutional principles. *Social Work, 40*(1), 55-64.

Anglin, D., Hser, Y., & Booth, M. W. (1987). Sex differences in addict careers: Vol. 4. Treatment. *American Journal of Drug and Alcohol Abuse, 13,* 253-280.

Baby fed crack dies: Mother is charged. (1995, October 5). *New York Times,* pp. A5, A27.

Barone, D. (1993). Wednesday's child: Literacy development of children prenatally exposed to crack/cocaine. *Research in the Teaching of English, 27,* 7-45.

Barone, D. (1994a, October). Myths about crack babies. *Educational Leadership, 52,* 67-68.

Barone, D. (1994b). The importance of classroom contacts: Literacy development of children prenatally exposed to crack/cocaine—Year 2. *Research in the Teaching of English, 28*(3), 286-311.

Barone, D. (1995). Be very careful not to let the facts get mixed up with the truth: Children prenatally exposed to crack/cocaine. *Urban Education, 30,* 40-55.

Barton, S. J., Harrigan, R., & Tse, A. M. (1995). Prenatal cocaine exposure: Implications for practice, policy, development, and needs for future reference. *Journal of Perinatology, 15,* 10-22.

Bateman, D. A., & Heagarty, M. C. (1989). Passive freebase cocaine (crack) inhalation by infants and toddlers. *American Journal of the Diseases of Children, 143*, 25-27.

Bateman, D. A., Ng, S. K. C., Hansen, C. A., & Heagarty, M. C. (1993). The effects of intrauterine cocaine exposure in newborns. *American Journal of Public Health, 83*, 190-193.

Bates, A. S., Fitzgerald, J. F., Dittus, R. S., & Wolinsky, F. D. (1994). Risk factors for underimmunization in poor urban infants. *Journal of the American Medical Association, 272*, 1105-1110.

Bauchner, H., Zuckerman, B., McClain, M., Frank, D., Fried, L., & Kayne, H. (1988). Risk of sudden infant death syndrome among infants with in utero exposure to cocaine. *Journal of Pediatrics, 113*, 831-834.

Beckman, L. J., & Amaro, H. (1984). Patterns of women's use of alcohol treatment agencies. In S. C. Wilsnack & L. J. Beckman (Eds.), *Alcohol problems in women* (pp. 319-348). New York: Guilford.

Belenko, S. R. (1993). *Crack and the evolution of anti-drug policy.* Westport, CT: Greenwood.

Besharov, D. (1989). The children of crack: Will we protect them? *Public Welfare 47*(4), 6-11.

Besharov, D. J. (1990). Crack children in foster care. *Children Today, 19*, 21-25, 35.

Bingol, N., Fuchs, M., Diaz, V., Stone, R., & Gromisch, D. (1987). Teratogenicity of cocaine in humans. *Journal of Pediatrics, 110*, 93-96.

Blakeslee, S. (1989, September 17). Crack's toll among babies: A joyless view, even of toys. *The New York Times*, p. A1.

Blejer, H. P. (1965, September). Coca leaf and cocaine addiction—Some historical notes. *Canadian Medical Association Journal, 25*, 702.

Blume, S. B. (1990). Chemical dependency in women: Important issues. *American Journal of Drug and Alcohol Abuse, 16*, 297-307.

Bowes, W. A., & Selgestad, B. (1981). Fetal versus maternal rights: Medical and legal perspectives. *Obstetrics and Gynecology, 58*, 209-214.

Breitbart, V., Chavkin, W., & Wise, P. (1994). The accessibility of drug treatment for pregnant women: A survey of programs in five cities. *American Journal of Public Health, 84*(10), 1658-1661.

Broekhuizen, F. F., Utrie, J., & Van Mullem, C. (1992). Drug use or inadequate prenatal care? Adverse pregnancy outcome in an urban setting. *American Journal of Obstetrics and Gynecology, 166*(6), 1747-1756.

Bureau of Narcotics. (1939). *Traffic in opium and other dangerous drugs.* Washington, DC: Government Printing Office.

Burkett, G., Yasin, S. Y., Palow, D., LaVoie, L., & Martinez, M. (1994). Patterns of cocaine binging: Effect on pregnancy. *American Journal of Obstetrics and Gynecology, 171*, 372-379.

Burt, M. R., Glynn, T. J., & Sowder, B. J. (1979). *Psychosocial characteristics of drug-abusing women.* Rockville, MD: National Institute on Drug Abuse.

Castelli, J. (1993). Unhealthy habits cost billions. Doctors fail to connect job to illness . . . Few know of alcohol's harm to fetus. *Safety and Health, 147*, 87-89.

Caughy, M., DiPietro, J. A., & Strobino, D. M. (1994). Day care participation as a protective factor in the cognitive development of low-income children. *Child Development, 65*(2), 457-471.

Center for Reproductive Law and Policy. (1993). Punishing women for their behavior during pregnancy: A public health disaster. *Reproductive Freedom in Focus*, 1-13.

Centers for Disease Control. (1991). *Preventing lead poisoning in young children: A statement by the Centers for Disease Control*. Atlanta, GA: U.S. Department of Health and Human Services, Public Health Service.

Chasnoff, I. J. (1986). *Drug use in pregnancy: Mother and child*. Lancaster, England: MTP.

Chasnoff, I. J. (1986/1987, Winter). Cocaine and pregnancy. *Childbirth Educator,* 37-42.

Chasnoff, I. J. (1987, May). Perinatal effects of cocaine. *Contemporary OB/GYN,* 163-179.

Chasnoff, I. J., Burns, W. J., Schnoll, S. H., & Burns, K. A. (1985). Cocaine use in pregnancy. *New England Journal of Medicine, 313,* 666-669.

Chasnoff, I. J., Chisum, G. M., & Kaplan, W. E. (1988). Maternal cocaine use and genitourinary tract malformations. *Teratology, 37,* 201-204.

Chasnoff, I. J., & Griffith, D. R. (1989a). Cocaine: Clinical studies of pregnancy and the newborn. In D. E. Hutchings (Ed.), *Prenatal abuse of licit and illicit drugs* (pp. 260-266). New York: Academy of Sciences.

Chasnoff, I. J., & Griffith, D. R. (1989b). Cocaine-exposed infants: Two year follow-up. *Pediatric Research, 25,* 249A.

Chasnoff, I. J., Griffith, D. R., Freier, C., & Murray, J. (1992). Cocaine/polydrug use in pregnancy: Two-year follow-up. *Pediatrics, 89,* 284-289.

Chasnoff, I. J., Griffith, D. R., MacGregor, S., Dirkes, K., & Burns, K. A. (1989). Temporal patterns of cocaine use in pregnancy. *Journal of the American Medical Association, 261,* 1741-1744.

Chasnoff, I. J., Landress, H. J., & Barrett, M. E. (1990). The prevalence of illicit drug or alcohol use during pregnancy and discrepancies in mandatory reporting in Pinellas County, Florida. *New England Journal of Medicine, 322,* 1202-1206.

Chasnoff, I. J., Lewis, D. E., & Squires, L. (1987). Cocaine intoxification in a breast-fed infant. *Pediatrics, 80,* 836-838.

Chasnoff, I. J., Schnoll, W. J., & Burns, K. A. (1986). Effects of cocaine on pregnancy outcome. *National Institute on Drug Abuse Research Monograph, Series, 7,* 335-341.

Chavkin, W. (1990). Drug addiction and pregnancy: Policy crossroads. *American Journal of Public Health, 80*(4), 483-487.

Cherukuri, R., Minkoff, H., Feldman, J., Parekh, A., & Glass, L. (1988). A cohort study of alkaloid cocaine ("crack") in pregnancy. *Obstetrics and Gynecology, 72,* 147.

Chira, S. (1990, May 25). Crack babies turn 5, and schools brace. *The New York Times,* pp. A1, B5.

Cisin, I., Miller, J. D., & Harrell, A. V. (1978). *Highlights from the National Survey on Drug Abuse 1977*. Rockville, MD: National Institute on Drug Abuse.

Cohen, S. (1984, April-June). Recent developments in the use of cocaine. *Bulletin on Narcotics, 9.*

Cole, C. D., & Platzman, K. A. (1993). Behavioral development in children prenatally exposed to drugs. *International Journal of the Addictions, 28*(13), 1393-1433.

Colen, B. D. (1990, April 23). Cocaine babies: Doctors are becoming increasingly alarmed about the long-term prospects for a growing army of damaged children. *News Monitor: Selected Articles of Interest in the Public Press,* 17-19.

Colten, M. E. (1979). A descriptive and comparative analysis of self-perceptions and attitudes of heroin-addicted women. In *Addicted women: Family dynamics, self perceptions, and support systems* (pp. 7-36). Rockville, MD: National Institute on Drug Abuse.

Condon, C. M. (1995). Clinton's cocaine babies. *Policy Review, 72,* 12-15.

Cuskey, W. R., Richardson, A. H., & Berger, L. H. (1979). *Specialized therapeutic community program for female addicts.* Rockville, MD: National Institute on Drug Abuse.

Dal Pazzo, E. E., & Marsh, F. H. (1987). Psychosis and pregnancy: Some new ethical and legal dilemmas for the physician. *American Journal of Obstetrics and Gynecology, 156*(2), 425-427.

Dickson, P. H., Lind, A., Studts, P., Nipper, H. C., Makoid, M., & Therkildsen, D. (1994). The routine analysis of breast milk for drug abuse in a clinical toxicology laboratory. *Journal of Forensic Sciences, 39*(1), 207-214.

DiPietro, J., Suess, P. E., Wheeler, J. S., Smouse, P. H., & Newlin, D. B. (1995). Reactivity and regulation in cocaine-exposed neonates. *Infant Behavior and Development, 18,* 407-414.

Dixon, S. D. (1994). Neurological consequences of prenatal stimulant drug exposure. *Infant Mental Health, 15*(2), 134-145.

Doberczak, T. M., Kandall, S. R., & Wilets, I. (1991). Neonatal abstinence syndrome in term and preterm infants. *Journal of Pediatrics, 118,* 933-937.

Dow-Edwards, D., Chasnoff, I. J., & Griffith, D. R. (1992). Cocaine use during pregnancy: Neurobehavioral changes in the offspring. In T. B. Sonderegger (Ed.), *Perinatal substance abuse: Research findings and clinical implications.* Baltimore: Johns Hopkins University Press.

Duncan, G., Brooks-Gunn, J., & Klebanov, P. (1994). Economic deprivation and early childhood development. *Child Development, 65,* 296-318.

Edmondson, R., & Smith, T. M. (1994). Temperament and behavior of infants prenatally exposed to drugs: Clinical implications for the mother-infant dyad. *Infant Mental Health Journal, 15*(4), 368-379.

Erickson, P. G., & Murray, G. F. (1989). Sex differences in cocaine use and experiences: A double standard revived? *American Journal of Drug and Alcohol Abuse, 15,* 135-152.

Ernst, A. A., Romolo, R., & Nick, T. (1993). Emergency department screening for syphilis in pregnant women without prenatal care. *Annals of Emergency Medicine, 22*(5), 781-785.

Ewing, H. (1992). Care of women and children in the perinatal period. In M. F. Fleming & K. L. Barry (Eds.), *Addictive disorders* (pp. 211-231). St. Louis: Mosby-Year Book.

Fackelman, K. (1991). The maternal cocaine connection: A tiny unwitting victim may bear the brunt of drug abuse. *Science News, 140,* 152.

Farr, K. A. (1995). Fetal abuse and the criminalization of behavior during pregnancy. *Crime & Delinquency, 41*(2), 235-245.

Feldman, H. W. (1968). Ideological supports to becoming and remaining a heroin addict. *Journal of Health Studies and Social Behavior, 9,* 131-139.

Fenton, L., McLaren, M., Wilson, A., Anderson D., & Curry, S. (1993). Prevalence of maternal drug use near time of delivery. *Connecticut Medicine, 57*(10), 655-659.

Fishel, R., Hamamoto, G., Barbul, A., Niji, V., & Efron, G. (1985). Cocaine colitis: Is this a new syndrome? *Colon and Rectum, 28,* 264-266.

Frank, D. A., Bauchner, H., Parker, S., Huber, A., Kyei-Aboagye, K., Cabral, H., & Zuckerman, B. (1990). Neonatal body proportionality and body composition after in utero exposure to cocaine and marijuana. *Journal of Pediatrics, 117,* 622-626.

Fried, P. A., & O'Connell, C. M. (1987). A comparison of the effects of prenatal exposure to tobacco, alcohol, cannabis, and caffeine on birth size and subsequent growth. *Neurobehavioral Toxicology and Teratology, 9,* 79-85.

Fried, P. A., & Watkinson, B. (1990). 36 and 48 month neurobehavioral follow-up of children prenatally exposed to marijuana, cigarettes, and alcohol. *Journal of Developmental and Behavioral Pediatrics, 11,* 49-58.

Fulroth, R. F., Durand, D. J., Nicjerson, B. G., & Espinoza, A. M. (1989). Prenatal cocaine exposure is not associated with a large increase in the incidence of SIDS. *Pediatric Research, 25,* 215A.

Fulroth, R. F., Phillips, B., & Durant, D. J. (1989). Perinatal outcome of infants exposed to cocaine and/or heroin in utero. *American Journal of Diseases in Children, 143,* 905-910.

Funkhouser, A. W., Butz, A. M., Feng, T. I., McCaul, M. E., & Rosenstein, B. J. (1993). Prenatal care and drug use in pregnant women. *Drug and Alcohol Dependence, 33,* 1-9.

Garcia, S. A., & Segalman, R. (1991). The control of perinatal drug abuse: Legal, psychological, and social imperatives. *Law and Psychology Review, 15,* 19-64.

Garrity-Rokous, F. E. (1994). Punitive legal approaches to the problem of prenatal drug exposure. *Infant Mental Health Journal, 15*(2), 218-237.

Gawin, F. H., & Ellinwood, E. H. (1988). Cocaine and other stimulants: Actions, abuse, and treatment. *New England Journal of Medicine, 318,* 1173-1182.

Golden, M. R. (1991). When pregnancy discrimination is gender discrimination: The constitutionality of excluding pregnant women from drug treatment programs. *New York University Law Review, 66,* 1832-1880.

Gomby, D. S., & Shiono, P. H. (1991). Estimating the number of substance-exposed infants. *The Future of Children, 1,* 17-25.

Gonzalez, N., & Campbell, M. (1994). Cocaine babies: Does prenatal exposure to cocaine affect development? *Journal of the American Academy of Child and Adolescent Psychiatry, 33,* 16-19.

The gourmet cokebook: A complete guide to cocaine. (1972). San Francisco: White Mountain.

Grabowski, J. (Ed.). (1984). *Cocaine: Pharmacology, effects, and treatment of abuse.* Rockville, MD: National Institute on Drug Abuse.

Greene, M. H. (1974). An epidemiologic assessment of heroin use. *American Journal of Public Health, 64*(Suppl.), 1-10.

Greenleaf, V. D. (1989). *Women and cocaine: Personal stories of addiction and recovery.* Los Angeles: Lowell House.

Gregorchik, L. A. (1992). The cocaine-exposed children are here. *Phi Delta Kappan, 73*(9), 709-711.

Greider, K. (1995, July/August). Crackpot ideas. *Mother Jones,* 53-56.

Griffin, M. L., Weiss, R. D., Mirin, S. M., & Lange, U. A. (1989, February). A comparison of male and female cocaine abusers. *Archives of General Psychiatry, 46,* 122-126.

Griffith, D. R., Azuma, S. D., & Chasnoff, I. (1994). Three-year outcome of children exposed prenatally to drugs. *Journal of the American Academy of Child and Adolescent Psychiatry, 33,* 20-27.

Handler, A., Kistin, N., Davis, F., & Ferre, C. (1991). Cocaine use during pregnancy: Perinatal outcomes. *American Journal of Epidemiology, 133,* 818-825.

Harrington, D., Dubowitz, H., Black, M. M., & Binder, A. (1995). Maternal substance use and neglectful parenting: Relations with children's development. *Journal of Clinical Child Psychology, 24*(3), 258-263.

Harrison, P. A. (1989). Women in treatment: Changing over time. *International Journal of the Addictions, 24,* 655-673.

Hawk, M. N. (1994). How social policies make matters worse: The case of maternal substance abuse. *Journal of Drug Issues, 24*(3), 517-526.

Hawley, T. L., Halle, T. G., Drasin, R. E., & Thomas, N. G. (1995). Children of addicted mothers: Effects of the crack epidemic on the caregiving environment and the development of preschoolers. *American Journal of Orthopsychiatry, 65*(3), 364-379.

Hawthorne, J. L., & Maier, R. C. (1993). Drug abuse in an obstetric population of a midsized city. *Southern Medical Journal, 86*(12), 1334-1338.

Hopkins, E. (1990, October 18). Childhood's end. *Rolling Stone,* 66.

Hospital gives up notifying police of cocaine abusers. (1994, September 8). *New York Times,* p. A18.

Hser, Y., Anglin, M. D., & Booth, M. W. (1987). Sex differences in addict careers: III. Addiction. *American Journal of Drug and Alcohol Abuse, 13,* 231-251.

Hunt, L. G., & Chambers, C. D. (1976). *The heroin epidemics.* New York: Spectrum.

Huston, A. C., McLoyd, V. C., & Coll, C. G. (1994). Children and poverty: Issues in contemporary research. *Child Development, 65,* 275-282.

Inciardi, J. A. (1992). *The war on drugs II: The continuing epic of heroin, cocaine, crack, crime, AIDS, and public policy.* Mountain View, CA: Mayfield.

Inciardi, J. A. (1996). Alcohol and drug use in prison. In *Encyclopedia of American Prisons* (pp. 168-170). New York: Macmillan.

Inciardi, J. A., Lockwood, D., & Pottieger, A. E. (1993). *Women and crack cocaine.* New York: Macmillan.

Jacobson, J. L., Jacobson, S. W., & Sokol, R. J. (1994). Effects of prenatal exposure to alcohol, smoking, and illicit drugs on postpartum somatic growth. *Alcoholism: Clinical and Experimental Research, 18,* 317-323.

Jacobson, J. L., Jacobson, S. W., Sokol, R. J., Martier, S. S., Ager, J. W., & Shankaran, S. (1994). Effects of alcohol use, smoking, and illicit drug use on fetal growth in black infants. *Journal of Pediatrics, 124,* 757-764.

Jaudes, P. K., Ekwo, E., & Van Voorhis, J. (1995). Association of drug abuse and child abuse. *Child Abuse & Neglect, 19*(9), 1065-1075.

Jones, E. (1953). *The life and work of Sigmund Freud* (Vol. 1). New York: Basic Books.

Jones, K. L., Smith, D. W., Ulleland, C. N., & Streissguth, A. P. (1973). Pattern of malformation in offspring of chronic alcoholic mothers. *Lancet, 1,* 1267-1271.

Jos, P. H., Marshall, M. F., & Perlmutter, M. (1995). The Charleston policy on cocaine use during pregnancy: A cautionary tale. *Journal of Law, Medicine, & Ethics, 23,* 120-128.

Justin, R. G., & Rosner, F. (1989). Maternal/fetal rights: Two views. *Journal of the American Medical Women's Association, 44*(3), 90-95.

Kahn, E. J. (1960). *The big drink: The story of Coca-Cola.* New York: Random House.

Kalant, O. J. (1980). Sex differences in alcohol and drug problems—Some highlights. In O. J. Kalant (Ed.), *Research advances in alcohol and drug problems, Vol. 5: Alcohol and drug problems in women* (pp. 1-24). New York: Plenum.

Kantrowitz, B., & Wingert, P. (1990, February 12). The crack children. *Newsweek,* 62-63.

Kearney, M. H., Murphy, S., & Rosenbaum, M. (1994). Mothering on crack cocaine: A grounded theory analysis. *Social Science and Medicine, 38*(2), 351-361.

Kerr, P. (1986, August 25). Babies of crack users fill hospital nurseries. *The New York Times,* p. B1.

Keyes, L. J. (1992). Rethinking the aim of the "war on drugs": States' roles in preventing substance abuse by pregnant women. *Wisconsin Law Review, 1,* 197-232.

Kharasch, S. J., Glotzer, D., Vinci, R., Weitzman, M., & Sargent, J. (1991). Unsuspected cocaine exposure in young children. *American Journal of the Development of Children, 145,* 204-206.

Kim, M., Checola, R. T., Noble, L. M., & Yoon, J. J. (1989). Cocaine and congenital malformations. *Pediatric Research Proceedings, 25*(Part 2), 77A.

King, P. (1992). Helping women helping children: Drug policy and future generations. *Milbank Quarterly, 69*(4), 595-621.

Koren, G., Graham K., Shear, H., & Einarson, T. (1989). Bias against the null hypothesis: The reproductive hazards of cocaine. *Lancet, 2,* 1440-1442.

Kumpfer, K. L. (1991). Treatment programs for drug abusing women. *The Future of Children, 1,* 50-60.

Langone, J. (1988, September 19). Crack comes to the nursery. *Time,* 85.

Larson, C. (1991, Spring). Overview of state legislative and judicial responses. In *Future of Children* (pp. 72-83). Los Altos, CA: David and Lucile Packard Foundation, Center for the Future of Children.

Lester, B. M., Corwin, M. J., Sepkowski, C., Seifer, R., Peuker, M., McLaughlin, S., & Golub, H. L. (1991). Neurobehavioral syndromes in cocaine-exposed newborn infants. *Child Development, 62,* 694-705.

Lester, B. M., & Tronick, E. Z. (1994). The effects of prenatal cocaine exposure and child outcome. *Infant Mental Health Journal, 15*(2), 107-119.

Lewis, K. (1991). Pathophysiology of prenatal drug-exposure: In utero, in the newborn, in childhood, and in agencies. *Journal of Pediatric Nursing, 6,* 185-190.

Lex, B. K. (1991). Some gender differences in alcohol and polysubstance users. *Health Psychology, 10,* 121-132.

Lieb, J. L., & Sterk-Elifson, C. (1995). Crack in the cradle: Social policy and reproductive rights among crack-using females. *Contemporary Drug Problems, 22,* 687-705.

Lockitch, G., Berry, B., Roland, E., Wadsworth, L., Kaikov, Y., & Mirhady, F. (1991). Seizures in a 10-week-old infant: Lead poisoning from an unexpected source. *Canadian Medical Association Journal, 145*(11), 1465-1468.

Macdonald, P. T., Waldorf, D., Reinarman, C., & Murphy, S. (1988). Heavy cocaine use and sexual behavior. *Journal of Drug Issues, 18,* 437-455.

MacGregor, S. N., Keith, L. G., Chasnoff, I. J., Rosner, M. A., Chisum, G. M., Shaw, P., & Minoque, J. P. (1987). Cocaine use during pregnancy: Adverse perinatal outcome. *American Journal of Obstetrics and Gynecology, 157,* 686-690.

Madden, R. G. (1993). State actions to control fetal abuse: Ramifications for child welfare practice. *Child Welfare, 72*(2), 129-140.

Maher, L. (1990). Criminalizing pregnancy—The downside of a kinder, gentler nation? *Social Justice, 17*(3), 111-135.

Malakoff, M. E., Mayes, L. C., & Schottenfeld, R. S. (1994). Language abilities of preschool children living with cocaine-using mothers. *American Journal on Addictions, 3*(4), 346-354.

March of Dimes. (1992). *Cocaine use during pregnancy: Public health information sheet.* White Plains, NY: National Organization of American Health.

Mariner, W., Glantz, L. H., & Annas, G. J. (1990). Pregnancy, drugs, and the perils of prosecution. *Criminal Justice Ethics, 9,* 30-41.

Marks, M. (1990, April 16). Kindergarten: Crack's next stop. *Miami Herald,* p. A1.

Mathias, R. (1995, January/February). NIDA survey provides first national data on drug use during pregnancy. *NIDA Notes,* 6.

Mayes, L. C. (1992). Prenatal cocaine exposure and young children's development. *Annals of the American Academy of Political and Social Sciences, 521,* 11-27.

Mayes, L. C., Bornstein, M. H., Chawarska, K., & Granger, R. H. (1995). Information processing and developmental assessments in 3-month-old infants exposed prenatally to cocaine. *Pediatrics, 95,* 539-545.

McGinnis, D. M. (1990). Prosecution of mothers of drug-exposed babies: Constitutional and criminal theory. *University of Pennsylvania Law Review, 139,* 505-539.

McNamara, D. (1989). New York City's crack babies. *The New York Doctor, 2*(7), 1.

Mentis, M., & Lundgren, K. (1995). Effects of prenatal exposure to cocaine and associated risk factors on language development. *Journal of Speech and Hearing Research, 38,* 1303-1318.

Mieczkowski, T. (1990). The accuracy of self-reported drug use: An evaluation and analysis of new data. In R. Weisheit (Ed.), *Drugs, crime, and the criminal justice system* (pp. 275-302). Cincinnati, OH: Anderson.

Morales, E. (1989). *Cocaine: White gold rush in Peru.* Tucson: University of Arizona Press.

National Center for Health Statistics. (1995, November 30). Births, marriages, divorces, and deaths for June 1995. *Monthly Vital Statistics Report, 44*(6). Hyattsville, MD: Public Health Service.

National Institute on Drug Abuse. (1989, November/December). High risk of cocaine, other drugs: Babies and mothers. *ADAMHA News, 3,* 12.

National Institute on Drug Abuse. (1994, October 17). New NIDA research suggests crack baby epidemic overblown. *Substance Abuse Letter, 3.*

Needleman, H. L., & Bellinger, D. (Eds.). (1994). *Prenatal exposure to toxicants: Developmental consequences.* Baltimore, Johns Hopkins University Press.

Neuspiel, D. R., & Hamel, S. C. (1991). Cocaine and infant behavior. *Journal of Developmental and Behavioral Pediatrics, 12,* 55-64.

Neuspiel, D. R., Markowitz, M., & Drucker, E. (1994). Intrauterine cocaine, lead, and nicotine exposure and fetal growth. *American Journal of Public Health, 84,* 1492-1495.

Newacheck, P., Jameson, W., & Halfon, N. (1994). Health status and income: The impact of poverty on child health. *Journal of School Health, 64,* 229-233.

Nicholl, C. (1985). *The fruit palace.* New York: St. Martin's.

Norris, M. (1991, July 1). And the children shall need. *Washington Post,* p. A1.

Novacek, J., Raskin, R., & Hogan, R. (1991). Why do adolescents use drugs? Age, sex, and user differences. *Journal of Youth and Adolescence, 20,* 475-492.

Nulman, I., Rovet, J., Altmann, D., Bradley, C., Einarson, T., & Koren, G. (1994). Neurodevelopment of adopted children exposed in utero to cocaine. *Canadian Medical Association Journal, 151*(11), 1591-1597.

Nurco, D. N., Wegner, N., Baum, H., & Makotsky, A. (1979). A case study: Narcotic addiction over a quarter of a century in a major American city 1950-1977. Rockville, MD: National Institute on Drug Abuse.

Okoruwa, E., Shah, R., & Gerdes, K. (1995). Apnea and vomiting in an infant due to cocaine exposure. *Journal of the Iowa Medical Society, 85*(11), 449-450.

Paltrow, L. (1992). *Criminal prosecutions against pregnant women: National update and overview.* New York: American Civil Liberties Union Foundation, Reproductive Freedom Project.

Partridge, E. (1961). *A dictionary of the underworld.* New York: Bonanza.

Peak, K., & Del Papa, F. S. (1993). Criminal justice enters the womb: Enforcing the "right" to be born drug-free. *Journal of Criminal Justice, 21,* 245-263.

Pinkney, D. S. (1989, October 6). Cocaine babies: Lifetime of challenge. *American Medical News,* 16-20.

Porat, R., Brodsky, N. L., Giannetta, J. M., & Hurt, H. (1994). Association of sudden infant death (SIDS) and in utero cocaine exposure: A controlled, prospective, blinded study. *Pediatric Research, 35*(4), 284A.

Posner, J. K., & Vandell, D. L. (1994). Low-income children's after school care: Are there beneficial effects of after school programs? *Child Development, 65*(2), 440-456.

Prather, J. E., & Fidell, L. S. (1978). Drug use and abuse among women: An overview. *International Journal of the Addictions, 13,* 863-885.

Preble, E., & Casey, J. J., Jr. (1969). Taking care of business: The heroin user's life on the street. *International Journal of the Addictions, 4,* 1-24.

Public Health Foundation. (1990, January/February). Cocaine-exposed babies may face impaired development. *Public Health Macroview,* 2.

Ramer, B. S., Smith, D. E., & Gay, G. R. (1972). Adolescent heroin abuse in San Francisco. *International Journal of the Addictions, 7,* 461-465.

Randall, T. (1991). "Intensive" prenatal care may deliver healthy babies to pregnant drug abusers. *Journal of the American Medical Association, 265*(21), 2773-2774.

Ratner, M. S. (Ed.). (1993). *Crack pipe as pimp: An ethnographic investigation of sex-for-crack exchanges.* New York: Lexington.

Reed, B. G. (1991). Linkages: Battering, sexual assault, incest, child sexual abuse, teen pregnancy, dropping out of school and the alcohol and drug connection. In P. Roth (Ed.), *Alcohol and drugs are women's issues: Vol. I. A review of the issues* (pp. 130-149). Metuchen, NJ: Women's Action Alliance and Scarecrow.

Revkin, A. C. (1989, September). Crack in the cradle. *Discover,* 62-69.

Richardson, G. A., & Day, N. L. (1994). Detrimental effects of prenatal cocaine exposure: Illusion or reality? *Journal of the American Academy of Child and Adolescent Psychiatry, 33*(1), 28-34.

Richardson, G., Day, N., & McGauhey, P. (1993). The impact of perinatal marijuana and cocaine use on the infant and child. *Clinical Obstetrics and Gynecology, 36,* 302-318.

Rist, M. C. (1990). "Crack babies" in school. *American School Board Journal, 177,* 19-24.

Robins, L. N., & Mills, J. L. (Eds.). (1993). Effects of in utero exposure to street drugs. *American Journal of Public Health, 83*(Suppl.), 1-32.

Rodriguez, M. (1989). Treatment of cocaine abuse: Medical and psychiatric consequences. In K. K. Redda, C. A. Walker, & G. Barnett (Eds.), *Cocaine, marijuana, designer drugs: Chemistry, pharmacology, and behavior* (pp. 97-111). Boca Raton, FL: CRC.

Rosecan, J. S., & Gross, B. F. (1986). Newborn victims of cocaine abuse. *Medical Aspects of Human Sexuality, 11,* 30-35.

Rosenbaum, M. (1981). *Women on heroin*. New Brunswick, NJ: Rutgers University Press.

Rosenbaum, R. (1987, February 15). Crack murder: A detective story. *New York Times Magazine*, pp. 29-33, 57, 60.

Rosenberg, N., Meert, K., Knazik, S. R., Yee, H., & Kauffman, R. E. (1991). Occult cocaine exposure in children. *American Journal of Diseases of Children, 145,* 1430-1432.

Rosner, F., Bennett, A. J., Cassell, E. J., Farnsworth, P. B., Landolt, A. B., Loeb, L., Numann, P. J., Ona, F. V., Risemberg, H. M., Sechzer, P. H., & Sordillo, P. P. (1989, February). Fetal therapy and surgery: Fetal rights versus maternal obligations. *New York State Journal of Medicine,* 80-84.

Rothman, S. (1991). New techniques may help cocaine babies. *U.S. Journal.*

Rotholz, D. A., Snyder, P., & Peters, G. (1995). A behavioral comparison of preschool children at high and low risk from prenatal cocaine exposure. *Education and Treatment of Children, 18*(1), 1-18.

Rudigier, A. F., Crocker, A. C., & Cohen, H. J. (1990). The dilemmas of childhood: HIV Infection. *Children Today, 19,* 26-29.

Sautter, R. (1992). Crack: Healing the children: Kappan special report. *Phi Delta Kappan, 74,* K1-K12.

Scherling, D. (1994). Prenatal cocaine exposure and childhood psychopathology: A developmental analysis. *American Journal of Orthopsychiatry, 64*(1), 9-19.

Schneider, J. W., Griffith, D. R., & Chasnoff, I. J. (1989). Infants exposed to cocaine in utero: Implications for developmental assessment and intervention. *Infants and Young Children, 2,* 25-36.

Scholl, T. O., Hediger, M. L., & Belsky D. H. (1994). Prenatal care and maternal health during adolescence and pregnancy: A review and meta-analysis. *Journal of Adolescent Health, 15,* 444-456.

Sexson, W. R. (1993). Cocaine: A neonatal perspective. *International Journal of the Addictions, 28*(7), 585-598.

Sherman, R. (1988, October 2). Keeping baby safe from mom. *National Law Journal, 1,* 24-25.

Shiono, P. H., Klebanoff, M. A., Nugent, R. P., Cotch, M. F., Wilkins, D. G., Rollins, D. E., Carey, J. C., & Behrman, R. E. (1995). The impact of cocaine and marijuana use on low birth weight and preterm birth: A multicenter study. *American Journal of Obstetrics and Gynecology, 172*(1), 19-27.

Silverman, N. S., Darby, M. J., Ronkin, S. L., & Wapner, R. J. (1991). Hepatitis B prevalence in an unregistered prenatal population: Implications for neonatal therapy. *Journal of the American Medical Association, 266*(20), 2852-2855.

Singer, L., Arendt, R., Minnes, S., Farkas, K., Yamashita, T., & Kliegman, R. (1995). Increased psychological distress in post-partum, cocaine-using mothers. *Journal of Substance Abuse, 7*(2), 165-174.

Singer, L., Arendt, R., Song, L. Y., Warshawsky, E., & Kliegman, R. (1994). Direct and indirect interactions of cocaine with childbirth outcomes. *Archives of Pediatric and Adolescent Medicine, 148,* 959-964.

Singh, G. K., & Yu, S. M. (1995). Infant mortality in the United States: Trends, differentials, and projections, 1950 through 2010. *American Journal of Public Health, 85*(7), 957-964.

Smith, G., & Dabiri, G. (1991). Prenatal drug exposure: The constitutional implications of three government approaches. *Constitutional Law Journal, 2,* 53-126.

Spears, R. A. (1981). *Slang and euphemism*. Middle Village, NY: Jonathan David.

Stevens, S., Arbiter, N., & Glider, P. (1989). Women residents: Expanding their role to increase treatment effectiveness in substance abuse programs. *International Journal of the Addictions, 24,* 425-434.

Stone, A. (1989, June 8). Crack babies born to life of suffering. *USA Today,* p. 3A.

Stone, N., Fromme, M., & Kogan, D. (1984). *Cocaine: Seduction and solution.* New York: Pinnacle.

Streissguth, A. P., Barr, H. M., Sampson, P. D., Darby, B. L., & Martin, D. C. (1989). IQ at age 4 in relation to maternal alcohol use and smoking during pregnancy. *Developmental Psychology, 25,* 3-11.

Suffet, F., & Brotman, R. (1976). Female drug use: Some observations. *International Journal of the Addictions, 11,* 19-33.

Sutter, A. G. (1966). The world of the righteous dope fiend. *Issues in Criminology, 2,* 177-222.

Terry, C. E., & Pellens, M. (1928). *The opium problem.* New York: Bureau of Social Hygiene.

Terry, D. (1996, August 17). In Wisconsin, a rarity of a fetal-harm case. *New York Times,* p. 6.

Thornton, J. (1988/1989, December 26-January 2). Ministering to the "Boarder Babies." *U.S. News and World Report,* 42-45.

Tomkins, A., & Kepfield, S. (1992). Policy responses when women use drugs during pregnancy: Using child abuse laws to combat substance abuse. In T. B. Sondregger (Ed.), *Perinatal substance abuse: Research findings and clinical implications.* Baltimore: Johns Hopkins University Press.

Toufexis, A. (1991, May 13). Innocent victims. *Time,* 56-60.

Tronick, E. Z., & Beeghly, M. (1992). Effects of prenatal exposure to cocaine on newborn behavior and development: A critical review. In *Identifying the needs of drug-affected children: Public policy issues* (OSAP Prevention Monograph 11). Rockville, MD: DHHS/PHS Office for Substance Abuse Prevention.

Trost, C. (1989, December 27). As drug babies grow older, schools strive to meet their needs. *Wall Street Journal,* p. A1.

U.S. Bureau of the Census. (1992). Poverty in the United States, 1991. *Current Population Reports* (Series P-60, No. 181). Washington, DC: Government Printing Office.

U.S. Department of Health and Human Services. (1994). Blood lead levels—United States, 1988-1991. *Morbidity and Mortality Weekly Report, 43,* 545-548.

van Baar, A. L., & de Graaff, B. M. T. (1994). Cognitive development at preschool-age of infants of drug-dependent mothers. *Developmental Medicine and Child Neurology, 36,* 1063-1075.

VandenBerg, K., Sweet, N., Weston, D., Fleisher, B. E., Johnson, A., & Stevenson, D. K. (1994, May). *Behavioral assessments of very low birth weight cocaine-exposed prematures differentiated them from non-exposed counterparts: Social interventions helped improve social outcomes.* Paper presented at the Annual Meeting of the American Pediatric Society, Seattle, WA.

Vandor, M., Juliana, P., & Leone, R. (1991). Women and illegal drugs. In P. Roth (Ed.), *Alcohol and drugs are women's issues: Vol. I. A review of the issues* (pp. 155-160). Metuchen, NJ: Women's Action Alliance and Scarecrow.

Van Dyke, D. C., & Fox, A. A. (1990). Fetal drug exposure and its possible implications for learning in the preschool and school-age population. *Journal of Learning Disabilities, 23,* 160-163.

Vimpani, G. (1995). Could your young patient have lead poisoning? *Australian Family Physician, 24,* 1446-1454.

Volpe, J. J. (1992). Effect of cocaine use on the fetus. *New England Journal of Medicine, 327*(6), 399-407.

Ward, S. L., Bautista, D. B., Schuetz, S., Wachsman, L., Bean, X., & Keens, T. G. (1989). Abnormal hypoxic arousal responses in infants of cocaine-abusing mothers. In D. E. Hutchings (Ed.), *Prenatal abuse of licit and illicit drugs: Annals of the New York Academy of Sciences.* New York: New York Academy of Sciences.

Wasserman, D. R., & Leventhal, J. M. (1993). Maltreatment of children born to cocaine-dependent mothers. *American Journal of Diseases of Children, 147,* 1324-1328.

Watkins, J., & Watkins, S. (1992). Prenatal drug exposure: The pro and con arguments for criminalizing fetal harm. *Journal of Crime and Justice, 15*(1), 157-172.

Weinstein, L. (1983). Reproductive and fetal rights: A philosophical ideal or practical necessity? *American Journal of Obstetrics and Gynecology, 147*(7), 848-849.

Weisman, G. (1993). Adolescent PTSD and developmental consequences of crack dealing. *American Journal of Orthopsychiatry, 63*(4), 553-561.

Weiss, R. D., Mirin, S. M., & Bartel, R. L. (1994). *Cocaine.* New York: American Psychiatric Press.

Wentworth, H., & Flexner, S. B. (1975). *Dictionary of American slang.* New York: Thomas Y. Crowell.

Williams, T. (1992). *Crack house: Notes from the end of the line.* Reading, MA: Addison-Wesley.

Wilsnack, S. C. (1984). Drinking, sexuality, and sexual dysfunction in women. In S. C. Wilsnack & L. J. Beckman (Eds.), *Alcohol problems in women* (pp. 189-227). New York: Guilford.

Woods, J. R., Plessinger, M. A., & Clark, K. E. (1987). Effect of cocaine on uterine blood flow and fetal oxygenation. *Journal of the American Medical Association, 257,* 957-961.

Yazigi, R. A., Odem, R. R., & Polakoski, K. L. (1991). Demonstration of specific binding of cocaine to human spermatozoa. *Journal of the American Medical Association, 266*(14), 1956-1959.

Zuckerman, B. (1991). Drug-exposed infants: Understanding the medical risk. *The Future of Children, 1,* 26-35.

Zuckerman, B. (1993). Developmental considerations for drugs- and AIDS-affected infants. In R. P. Barth, J. Pietrzak, & M. Ramler (Eds.), *Families living with drugs and HIV* (pp. 37-58). New York: Guilford.

Name Index

Subject Index

About the Authors

James A. Inciardi, PhD, is Director of the Center for Drug and Alcohol Studies at the University of Delaware, Professor in the Department of Sociology and Criminal Justice at Delaware, Adjunct Professor in the Department of Epidemiology and Public Health at the University of Miami School of Medicine, and a Distinguished Professor at the State University of Rio de Janeiro in Brazil. Dr. Inciardi received his doctorate in sociology at New York University and has research, clinical, field, and teaching experience in the areas of AIDS, substance abuse, and criminal justice. He has done extensive consulting work nationally and internationally and has published 40 books and more than 200 articles and chapters in the areas of substance abuse, criminology, criminal justice, history, folklore, social policy, AIDS, medicine, and law.

Christine A. Saum, MA, is Research Associate in the Center for Drug and Alcohol Studies at the University of Delaware, working on studies of treatment barriers for cocaine-dependent women, treatment evaluation, and HIV/AIDS. She received her master's degree from the University of Florida and has authored numerous publications in the areas of substance abuse, treatment evaluation, and drug policy.

Hilary L. Surratt, MA, is Research Associate in the Comprehensive Drug Research Center at the University of Miami School of Medicine; the Project Director of an HIV/AIDS seroprevalence and prevention study in Rio de Janeiro, Brazil; and Project Director of a multisite female condom study. Both projects are funded by the National Institute on Drug Abuse. She received her master's degree from the University of Florida and has authored numerous publications in the areas of AIDS, substance abuse, and drug policy.